T0150108

MEDITATION FOR THE REST OF US

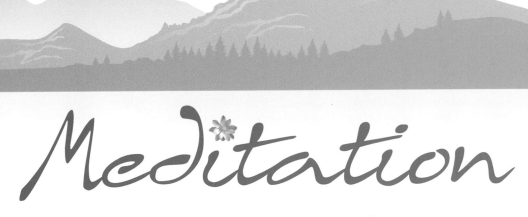

Meditation

for the Rest of Us

JAMES BALTZELL, MD

Fairview Press

MINNEAPOLIS

Fairview Press is a division of Fairview Health Services, a community-focused health system, affiliated with the University of Minnesota, providing a complete range of services, from the prevention of illness and injury to care for the most complex medical conditions. For a free catalog of Fairview Press titles, call toll-free 1-800-544-8207, or visit our website at www.fairviewpress.org.

The Center for Spirituality and Healing
Recognized nationally as a leader in integrative therapies and healing practices, the University of Minnesota Center for Spirituality & Healing's mission is to transform healthcare through innovative educational offerings, rigorous scientific research, and inspiring outreach programs.

Library of Congress Cataloging-in-Publication Data
Baltzell, James, 1950-
[Why meditation works]
Meditation for the rest of us / James Baltzell.
      p. cm.
    Originally published: Why meditation works. London : Polair Pub., 2006.
    ISBN-13: 978-1-57749-191-0 (pbk. : alk. paper)
    ISBN-10: 1-57749-191-2 (alk. paper)
  1. Meditation--Therapeutic use. 2. Meditation--History. I. Title.
    RC489.M43B35 2009
    616.89'16--dc22
                          2009003911

Printed in China
First printing: May 2009
13   12   11   10   09   7   6   5   4   3   2   1

Cover and book design by Ryan Scheife, Mayfly Design (www.mayflydesign.net)

Medical Disclaimer:
This publication is designed to provide accurate and authoritative information in regard to the subject matter covered. It is sold with the understanding that the publisher is not engaged in the provision or practice of medical, nursing, or professional healthcare advice or services in any jurisdiction. If medical advice or other professional assistance is required, the services of a qualified and competent professional should be sought. Neither Fairview Press nor the author is responsible or liable, directly or indirectly, for any form of damages whatsoever resulting from the use (or misuse) of information contained in or implied by these documents.

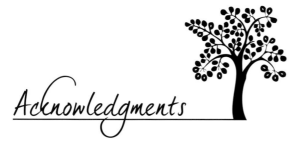

Acknowledgments

I should like to thank my wife Kärin for her patience while the book was written. Her excellent help and guidance are deeply appreciated. An additional thank you goes to Colum Hayward, my editor, who helped set up the book and then offered some very valuable suggestions to improve its flow.

I thank also Gaye Mack, a friend and author who contributed excellent ideas for the book, and to Esther Eichelberger who was a co-teacher of meditation for many years. She has helped develop many of the ideas about meditation.

Thanks go to the many meditation teachers, both seen and unseen, who have helped me over the years.

To my parents Virginia and Winston, I give thanks for the excellent education that helped form the basis for this book.

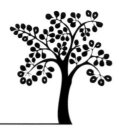

Contents

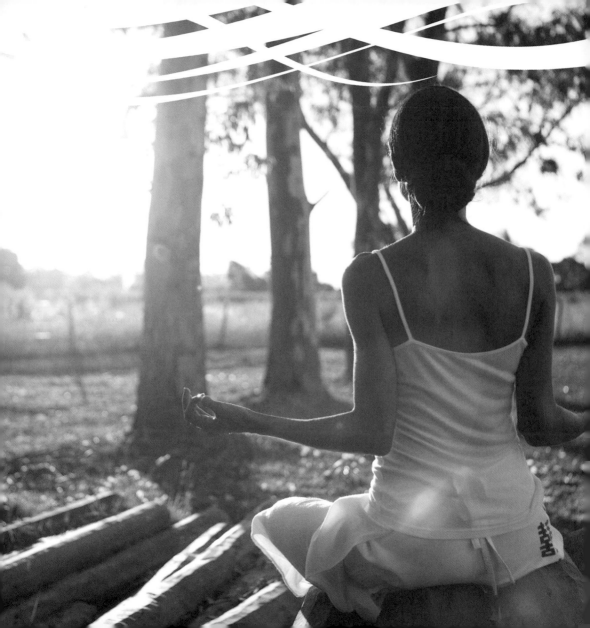

An Introduction to Meditation

MEDITATION IS BECOMING MAINSTREAM, enriching and improving lives. Meditation can be simple, as it takes only a few minutes to learn the basics, or it can be intricate, taking a lifetime to perfect. Moreover, its use is global. Most cultures and religions use meditation in some form.

Newsweek magazine reported on a poll of 1,004 adults by Princeton Survey Research Associates taken between August 2 and 4, 2005.[1] Among responders who had a daily spiritual or religious practice, 29 percent meditated. As an M.D. who meditates and teaches meditation, I have found the ability to meditate to be universal, with common scientific, religious, and spiritual aspects. There are both religious and non-religious forms of meditation.

The Asian traditions of Yoga, Hinduism, Buddhism, and Taoism have made meditation central to their teaching and have accumulated a vast body of knowledge about it. The Western cultures and religions, including Christianity, Judaism, and Islam, also have extensive knowledge about meditation. It would seem there are as many ways to meditate as there are ways to the top of

---

1   *Newsweek*, August 29, 2005, 48-9.

the mountain. How do we make sense of such a complex subject? Fortunately, we have knowledge from the great religions gleaned over the centuries, even though the subject of meditation stands independent of belief. This knowledge is now being combined with new scientific research.

It is my hope that after reading this book you, as a reader, will have a good basic understanding of meditation, how it works, the styles of meditation, and how to start meditating. This book will help to clarify meditation and give you a foundation to help you choose a meditation class.

Stress is commonly understood to cause many diseases. This connection will be explored in this book, highlighting the results of new research. New investigation is being done on the connection between the brain, the nervous system, the immune system, and stress. This study is called psychoneuroimmunology, or PNI. How we think does affect the body by way of the nerves, the hormones, and the immune system. Meditation is a tool that has been scientifically proven to lower the effects of stress, both by triggering what is known as the relaxation response (a physiological phenomenon) and also by accessing, in a positive way, the PNI system.

An interesting number of very recent, scientifically proven facts about meditation will also be discussed in this book. This is partly because medical equipment is now available that can detect the effects of meditation on the brain and the rest of the body.

As you will see in the next chapter, meditation works in three areas, the first of which has to do with relaxation of the body, the second with understanding the mind, and the third with spiritual awareness. You can access each or all of these, as you prefer. As you come in contact with the inner mind or inner self that is hidden by the noise of daily living, you may find you are able to be more intuitive and creative. Eventually—with time and practice—it is possible to reach a place of deep peace and calm. It is in this state that many feel closer to a higher power. With experience, you can achieve this calm state.

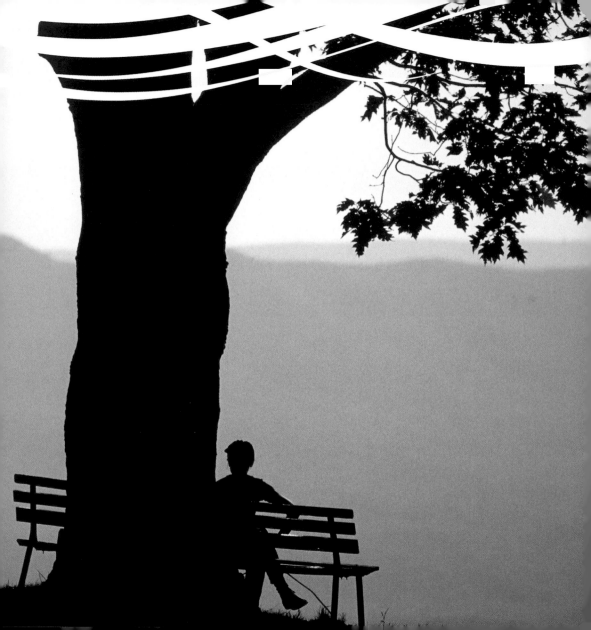

What is Meditation?

Meditation, according to a medical dictionary, is "a state of consciousness in which the individual eliminates environmental stimuli from awareness so that the mind can focus on a single thing, producing a state of relaxation and relief from stress. A wide variety of techniques are used to clear the mind of stressful outside interferences. It includes meditation therapy."[2]

The word "meditation" has a long history. It comes via French from the Latin *meditor*, which simply means "to think, consider, reflect upon." The initial syllable *med-*, along with *mod-*, is an ancient Indo-European component with the sense of "measure." The Sanskrit root of the word is *madha*, which means "wisdom." Hence it is also allied to verbs like "moderate" and "mediate"—not to mention adjectives such as "mid-" and "medial."

For ease of understanding, I have divided meditation into three stages. This is a simplistic way to describe and clarify an unseen and complex skill. Although I shall periodically use the word "stage," the stages are not sequential, and neither is one more "advanced" than another. They do represent choices, however,

---

2   *Mosby's Medical, Nursing, and Allied Health Dictionary.*

and you can choose to meditate at one, two, or three levels, or to go on to another stage at a later time. The only reason for putting them in the order that I have is that for many, the meditation path leads in that direction.

*The first stage of meditation is **physiological**: the process of relaxing and achieving the relaxation response.*

*The second stage is **insightful**: gaining knowledge of the inner self.*

*The third stage is **spiritual**: becoming aware of a higher consciousness and the spiritual world, and working in that world.*

Meditation is a key, a very important key, to your personal world. After calming the mind, meditation is listening, observing, and learning about your body, your mind, and the inner spiritual world. You move beyond everyday life and expand your awareness and consciousness.

Meditation can enrich your life as you learn about yourself and explore your inner world. Before you meditate, the everyday world seems to be black and white. After practicing meditation, you may find the world can be observed in living Technicolor. You can learn to be mindful of the present world, to let the past go, and to not worry about the future. You can learn how connected you are to others. This understanding can lead you to compassion and love for the world. What a great place this world would be if we could all practice love and compassion!

The ability to meditate is universal, with training. Hundreds of books have been written about meditation. There are many definitions of meditation, depending on the culture and religion of the writer. As far as this book is concerned, the word "meditation" is used to describe a person meditating on nature just as well as one who meditates for days in a religious order.

Examples of meditation include:

1. A few moments of quiet contemplation in a religious setting.
2. A person saying the Catholic rosary.
3. Quiet, attentive listening to music, or contemplating art or nature.
4. An athlete wholly in the moment in his or her sport.
5. A fisherman or woman quietly watching the water.
6. A person performing the conscious act of repetition of a word or mantra.
7. Mindfulness or insight meditation as practiced by a Buddhist.
8. Yoga, tai chi, or qi gong movement meditation.
9. Visualization meditation.
10. Deep spiritual meditation.
11. Repeating an affirmation.
12. Communion.

There are many different types of meditation, each of which may have different effects. Some of these effects are easy to measure: the effect on blood pressure, pulse, and breathing, to name a few. There is new scientific research on the measurable effects of meditation, the results of which will be explored later. Some effects are very difficult to understand, as they happen on an inner level. In the past, there have only been firsthand reports by experienced meditators to rely on. We shall explore the new research being done on the effects of meditation on the brain, as measured by Electroencephalography (EEG), Positive Emission Tomography (PET), Single Photon Emission Commuted Tomography (SPECT), Angiography, Computed Tomography (CT) and functional Magnetic Resonance Imaging (fMRI) machines.

There are common threads between the different types of meditation. Humans all have to deal with virtually the same body and mind, no matter which culture or religion they belong to. When people talk about meditation, it is like the blind men describing the elephant. One talks about the legs, another the trunk, and yet another the tail. Now it is possible to understand the common patterns in meditation and make better sense out of the different teachings. This understanding has been greatly facilitated now that teachings from around the world are open to public research.

Members of nearly all the Western religions, including Christianity, Judaism, and Islam, have practiced meditation throughout the centuries. In the list above, I mentioned reciting a rosary or chanting a mantra as types of meditation. Many have practiced quiet contemplation of God or the Divine. Although the Western religions have practiced meditation, it has not been as important as prayer. Prayer to God for help, forgiveness, or salvation is very important with the Western religions.

The Eastern systems largely teach that each person has to improve him or herself. Buddhist studies stress that the practitioner should work through meditation to be free of personal karma rather than appeasing a judgmental God. Meditation is very important for the Eastern traditions, particularly Buddhism, Hinduism, Yoga, and Taoism, which together have thousands of years of meditation history. Through meditation, the practitioners have learned about themselves, and with this knowledge they have achieved spiritual growth. Many of the Eastern traditions teach that by letting go of negative ideas such as fear, jealousy, attachment, and anger, you can be free to move to a state of love, free of attachment to the things of the world, and eventually move to a blissful state known as *nirvana*.

The Eastern traditions have many types of meditation. The most common methods involve either sitting or special forms of movement. Moving meditation is done in the yoga, tai chi, and qi gong[3] traditions. The meditation occurs while doing the postures or movements. Sitting meditation is also used.

---

3   Tai chi and qi gong are the most commonly seen transliterations of the Chinese names. Consistency would see either *taijiquan* alongside *qigong,* or *chi kung* alongside *tai chi.* The word *chi* or *qi* means the life force or essential energy.

Humans can meditate without training. This has been reported in a study by Mihaly Csikszentmihalyi.[4] There are many meditative moments during the day. There are also well-formalized methods of meditation that do not have religious connection. Repeating a word such as "one" will itself allow the participant to trigger the relaxation response and meditate. No religious connection is necessary.

We shall consider the relaxation response further in due course. It owes its name to Dr. Herbert Benson, of the Harvard Medical School, and was identified in his book, *The Relaxation Response*, as long ago as 1975. Benson discovered that all human beings are capable of the relaxation response. Visualization meditation and mindful meditation can also be done without religious connotations.[5]

My earlier distinction between three stages or types of meditation now needs further elaboration. The first is to relax the body and still the mind using a focus, like the breath, an object, a flame, or visualization. This can be done by anyone, with practice. There are great health benefits in this practice, including reduced stress and anxiety. During this stage the physiological relaxation response is activated.

---

4   *Flow: The Psychology of Optimal Experience.*

5   See, for instance, Shakti Gawain, *Creative Visualization*, and Jon Kabat-Zinn, *Full Catastrophe Living.*

The second is to work with and learn about your mind. The mind is very complex, with many levels. Some meditators have spent their whole lives meditating and learning about the mind. There are many modern teachers that can help us to understand this technique. This type of meditation is popular with many meditators including Buddhists and yogis, and is called the path of insight, or *vipassana* meditation. You can observe and name the ideas that come up in your mind, thereby gaining insight about your mind. This type of meditation has been combined with modern psychotherapy with excellent results.

The third element is that of moving to a higher consciousness. It is not necessary to go to this level when meditating, but people who do meditate for some time can have experiences that could be called spiritual. You can move beyond observation of your everyday thoughts to a spiritual reality or dimension. This is difficult to describe to the non-meditator. You have begun by settling down the body, then looking at the mind. Then what happens?

It appears there are similar experiences that have been reported by meditators the world over. These experiences have nonetheless been described in the context of each religion, culture, or type of meditation.

Some reported examples of what may happen in spiritual meditation include:

1. A feeling of peace and calm.
2. Sensing a switch from daily thoughts to a new, limitless space.

3. Awareness of being loved by a greater being, maybe seen as God.

4. Having knowledge of spiritual beings.

5. Contacting loved ones who have died and moved to the "other side."

6. Feeling love in the heart, mind, and body.

7. Awareness of energy moving through the body or up the spine.

8. Understanding that there is a connection with the rest of the world.

These occurrences and many others have been reported. Coming in contact with the spiritual reality is very meaningful on a personal level. People report a stronger faith after meditation.

Practitioners of many different religions have worshipped and loved a higher being. Mystics (a mystic might be described as one who, through special knowledge, has a direct awareness of the ultimate reality) from varied traditions have described a mystical state where there can be worship and communion with this higher being. The path of meditation is a special version of the path of devotion and it is used by Judaism, Christianity, Islam, and some forms of Hinduism. Personal contact in meditation and prayer with a higher spiritual reality can be very meaningful.

Some meditation schools train people to work on the higher levels to do healing for people and the world.[6] There are several methods for doing this. One is to send out love to the world from your heart. Another is to elevate yourself to the spiritual world in meditation and send out the healing from there. Symbols and colors are sometimes used.

The writer Stephan Bodian describes six levels of spiritual meditation: "believing in spirit, awakening to spirit, being in touch with spirit, being infused with spirit, being one with spirit, and no separation between spirit and ordinary life." He goes on to say, "When you meditate, you're bridging the apparent chasm that separates you, and connecting with your breath, with your body and senses, with your heart, with the present moment, and ultimately with a greater reality."[7]

In the past, it was necessary to retire from the world, be a monk, and spend one's whole life meditating or in contemplation to achieve the spiritual realm. Now there are other ways you can have the spiritual experience without retiring from society, although it still takes commitment and time.

Meditation is more effective, and can have more power, when done in a group. A leader can help guide your meditation. The combined power of thought

---

6   An example is the White Eagle Lodge, in Liss, Hampshire (UK).

7   *Meditation for Dummies*, 221-2

is said to give a stronger meditation. Jesus said, "Wherever two or three are gathered together in my name, there am I in the midst of them."[8]

Many artists and musicians have used meditation to release their creativity and intuition. Becoming aware of the beauty of the spiritual world can help you to create beauty in the everyday world.

Now, what is meditation? It is a means to learn about you—your physical, mental, and spiritual self. It can be a lifelong endeavor with many positive results, or it can be done over a short time to achieve a particular goal. You are free to meditate as long and as deeply as you wish, or to do it while you are walking, or to sit in the lotus position, or indeed in any position at all.

MEDITATION VERSUS PRAYER

Prayer, which can be viewed as supplication, is asking for help. Prayer acknowledges a higher power to which an appeal for help is made.

Meditation is relaxing, observing, and then most importantly listening and being aware of the inner voice, sometimes referred to as "the still voice."

It is possible both to pray and to meditate at the same sitting. With experience and practice, it is possible also to do both during daily life. If there is a

---

8   Matt. 18:20.

problem, a difficult task, or a need for creativity, it is possible to pray and appeal for help and guidance for the challenge ahead. However, it is not enough to pray for help. You also need to be quiet, be aware, and listen for inspiration. Help can come in many ways. You can feel stronger and more secure after a moment of relaxation and quiet time or you may find that new ideas come into your mind and your memory improves.

THINGS TO REMEMBER:

1. There are three levels on which you can practice meditation: physical, mental, and spiritual.

2. Meditation is a universal ability practiced with or without a religious connection.

3. Prayer is asking, and meditation is listening.

4. Meditation is a key to the inner world.

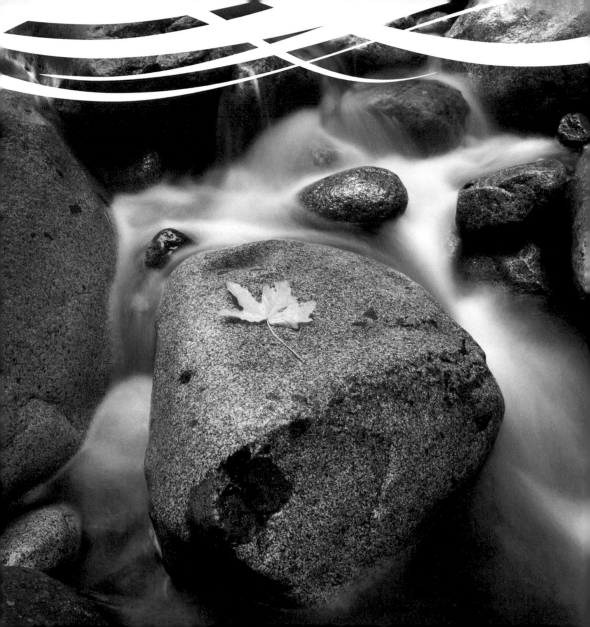

The History of Meditation

MEDITATION HAS MOST LIKELY been practiced in some form almost since human consciousness began. Indigenous people around the world have a long history of Shamanism, which uses a form of meditation (within the broad definition I have chosen). The holy person, sacred person, or medicine man or woman was able to reach a spiritual realm and receive answers for the tribe. The ability to meditate, at least in a basic way, appears to be an innate human ability. In 1995, I was lucky enough to have an interview with a wise woman of the Ojibwa, a Native American tribe. Like many modern medicine women, she was still able to describe a spiritual world similar to the one mentioned by other traditions and accessed through a form of meditation.

Each culture has used its own language to describe the techniques and effects of meditation. Many techniques were and are primitive; however, many are advanced and have been developed over the centuries. Once, religions taught meditation to disciples, keeping the techniques secret. Only after a time of training, testing, and initiation were these secrets revealed. It is only in the last century or so that most meditation techniques have become available worldwide. Some are still secret today.

Asia has been considered by many to be the birthplace of formal meditation. India and China appear to have a history of meditation dating back at least to 2500 BCE. There are figures in the lotus position on early artifacts that suggest someone meditating. By the time the Buddha came on the scene in the fourth, fifth, or sixth century BCE (scholarship varies), meditation was already a practice that was taught.

Both Hinduism and Buddhism have meditation and the study of meditation as an important part of their practices. At its spiritual level, yoga is defined as union, union between a person and the absolute. It is a meditation practice that originated very early in the Hindu tradition in India, and in its many branches it teaches both sitting and movement meditation. Yoga therapy, the postures that form part of the main tradition, is also used in medicine, and has proven very effective in correcting physical and mental ailments. Yoga is practiced all over the world and was brought to the Western world in the nineteenth century by Indian yogis and the Westerners who learned from them in India.

Among the many different types of yoga that are practiced, *hatha yoga*, very popular in the West, uses physical postures to bring the body into alignment. The movements and poses of *hatha yoga* can be done meditatively. *Raja yoga* and *mantra yoga*, as well as several other types, use sitting meditation. Yogis believe that both movement and sitting meditation will allow a healthy flow of energy through the body and the chakras (energy centers). If the practice of yoga is followed over many years, then *samadhi*, a super-conscious state or trance, can be reached.

Yogis are very knowledgeable about the effect of different types of breathing on the body. The respected teacher B. K. S. Iyengar has a particularly helpful book on the subject.[9] Students of yoga meditate extensively on the breath and the different ways to control the breath. This practice is called *pranayama*, control of the breath. They believe that *prana* is the life force, and that when you breathe correctly you bring this life force into your body. They believe *prana* will strengthen and heal your body. Many yogis spend one hour daily doing *pranayama* breathing and then do *hatha yoga* postures for several more hours. After this they will do sitting meditation. Most people only do *hatha yoga* postures or sitting meditation, or both. *Pranayama* is mostly done by more dedicated yogis.

Transcendental Meditation (TM) is a yogic practice and is very popular. It was developed by Maharishi Mahesh Yogi. He taught the use of a focus—in this case a word—as a mantra. TM begins with initial classes where the student receives his or her personal mantra (word). In meditation, the mantra is repeated over and over, eventually stilling the mind and relaxing the body. TM teaches that with time and the extensive practice of meditation, transcendental consciousness can be achieved. TM can be practiced independently of a re-

---

9   It is called *Light on Pranayama*. Readers wanting a shorter introduction may prefer Jenny Beeken's *Don't Hold Your Breath*, which is uniform with this volume.

ligion. There are centers around the world and a "university" in Fairfield, Iowa. Considerable meditation research has been performed by TM practitioners.

The Himalayan Institute is another meditation organization that is also based on the yogic tradition. It has many centers and is particularly popular in the United States. At the Institute, both movement and sitting meditation are taught, while ayurvedic medicine, a form of yogic medicine practiced for centuries in India, is also offered.

There are probably many thousands of Buddhist centers around the world that teach meditation. They differ in their teachings and traditions but have in common the teachings of the Buddha, the "awakened one." Following what Buddha taught, the tradition suggests that it is possible to have freedom from suffering through hard work, meditation, and love for all beings.[10] Buddha is not considered a God or even a representative of God by most Buddhists, but an enlightened teacher. The Buddha himself did not claim to believe in a personal God who demanded worship or who could offer salvation. Rather, he taught that spiritual growth comes through individual work. There are karmic debts (deeds from the past) that you need to expunge. The path to salvation therefore comes through your deeds and intentions, not through asking for forgiveness from God. Buddhists sometimes say "chop wood and carry water" to explain their method of living.

---

10   Pankaj Mishra's book *An End to Suffering* is a recent and particularly useful addition to books about Buddha.

Buddhists teach many ways to meditate, including mindful, insight, and loving-kindness meditations. Zen is a branch a little different from the others, whose mental practices help to teach us that words and sentences have no fixed meaning, and that logic as we understand it is often irrelevant.

Mindful meditation is bringing concentrated awareness to the breath, objects, or visualizations. Insight meditation (*vipassana*) is being aware of and observing thoughts in a non-attached way. It can help you to understand, "Who am I?" Insight meditation is frequently incorporated into modern psychotherapy and is helping to speed the therapeutic process. It is a very powerful technique allowing you to observe your thoughts and understand your innermost self.

Loving-kindness meditation helps you to love yourself and then send that love to the rest of the world. With loving-kindness meditation you learn great compassion for all living beings without discrimination, and to work for good, happiness, and peace. Buddhists have a wonderful meditation for sending love to the world.[11]

Many Buddhist and yogic meditators refer to a higher spiritual consciousness that can be encountered during meditation. For instance, they describe devas (equivalent to Christian angels) that can be seen when meditating. Others describe expanding the self until the self becomes one with spirit. Many of

---

11   A simple version is given as Visualization Three in Chapter Seven, "Sample Meditations."

them have used the advanced technique of chanting to achieve these higher levels of consciousness.

Taoism started in China at about the same time as Hinduism in India. Taoists learn nonviolence and meditation. Out of it came tai chi and qi gong, both of which are regarded as movement meditation. It is believed that performing the movements will help the practitioner achieve calm and eventually move him or her into deeper meditation. Tai chi and qi gong are techniques that are used to move and balance energy in the body.

Within Islam there is a meditative and esoteric branch, the Sufis, who meditate and practice *zikr*, the remembrance of the divine. There are many forms of *zikr*, ranging from silent meditations to enthusiastic dances. The ecstasy of the whirling dervishes is perhaps the most remarkable form of movement meditation to witness. The *zikr* can be done quietly meditating on a ring of beads similar to the Catholic rosary. The meditation can be short or last for hours. It is meant to open the heart to the divine all through the day.

The Jewish religion, too, has a mystical strand within it, the one that follows the teachings of the Kabbalah. Practitioners date their history back possibly to Abraham. For a long time they were a secret group that did not share their practices with the public. They have had a meditation tradition allowing them to work on the spiritual planes. Teaching and practice of the Kabbalah is currently widespread, with some famous converts, including Madonna.

Christians are especially known for their tradition of prayer for salvation. Yet they also have a history of meditation. There are many references to meditation in the Bible. Psalm 46 reads: "Be still and know that I am God." Paul commanded Timothy to "meditate on these things,"[12] while Joshua was charged by God to meditate day and night.[13] There have been many Christian mystics: Mother Julian of Norwich, Hildegard of Bingen, Jakob Boehme, St. Francis of Assisi, St. Teresa of Avila, and George Fox (the Quaker) are a few among many. Through prayer and meditation Christians can learn about an awakening of the light, or awakening the Christ spirit within the heart. This concept of light within the heart is also taught by most other religions.

Recently there has been a tendency to combine Eastern and Western techniques of prayer and meditation. People are finding out what works for them from all of the traditions and incorporating these practices into their lives. Because there is an inner desire for closeness with God, a study of meditation and the practice of meditation are beginning to be more widespread in the Christian churches. For example, *Newsweek* magazine reports[14] that two Trappist monks, Father Thomas Keating and Father William Meninger, "began teaching a form of Christian meditation that grew into the worldwide phenomenon known as centering prayer. Twice a day for twenty minutes,

---

12   1 Tim. 4:15.

13   Josh. 1:8.

14   Adler, J., "In Search of the Spirtual," *Newsweek*, August 29, 2005, 49.

practitioners find a quiet place to sit with their eyes closed and surrender their minds to God…. Keating is spreading the word to 'hungry people, looking for a deeper relationship with God.'" In the same article, a poll by Beliefnet, largely in the USA, reported that 57 percent of the respondents said spirituality was very important in their lives, and 27 percent said it was somewhat important. This adds up to 84 percent who thought spirituality was important! Most responded that you could go to heaven even if you followed another religion, implying that the consensus is that it is the way you live your life, combined with your relationship with God, which decides what happens to you in the afterlife.

There is a real search for God today, for a personal God with whom you can have a personal relationship. This search is leading people around the world to meditation as well as prayer. In the past, the priests or ministers provided the contact with God. Now many are not satisfied with worship at a distance and want a personal relationship. Because of this combination of Eastern, New Age, and Christian beliefs, a new yet old way to reach God is becoming mainstream.

Many other groups have used the combination of Eastern and Western meditation to reach higher spiritual levels. Non-denominational Christian meditation groups practice effective meditation methods that include imagery and guided meditations. The Spiritualists, the Theosophical Society, Rudolph Steiner's Anthroposophical Society, and the White Eagle Lodge are the longest-established among a great many that teach meditation. They teach a method of meditation that emphasizes light and love in the heart. They are also leaders in teaching spiritual meditation. Communication with spiritual beings and loved ones that have passed on to the other side are reported to occur with some meditations.

Non-religious groups also teach meditation. A non-religious form was popularized by Herbert Benson, M.D., the author of *The Relaxation Response*. There are many other types, such as the method taught by Shakti Gawain. (See p. 10.) Meditation is also now taught in medical settings to reduce pain, anxiety, and stress. It has been shown that meditation can be healing and help prevent disease. Meditation and psychotherapy are also being used together very effectively.

There are many famous medical centers that use meditation in the treatment of patients, including, in the United States, centers at Harvard, the University of Massachusetts, and the University of California, San Francisco. Meditation is slowly being accepted in medicine, particularly by practitioners of complementary medicine, as the author Gaye Mack describes in another book in this series, *Making Complementary Therapies Work for You*.

THINGS TO REMEMBER:

1. Meditation predates recorded history.

2. There are writings about meditation in almost all of the major religious traditions.

3. Meditation is widely used to achieve a connection with a higher power.

4. Meditation is helpful to improve mental and physical health.

5. Meditation is practiced by both non-religious and religious groups alike.

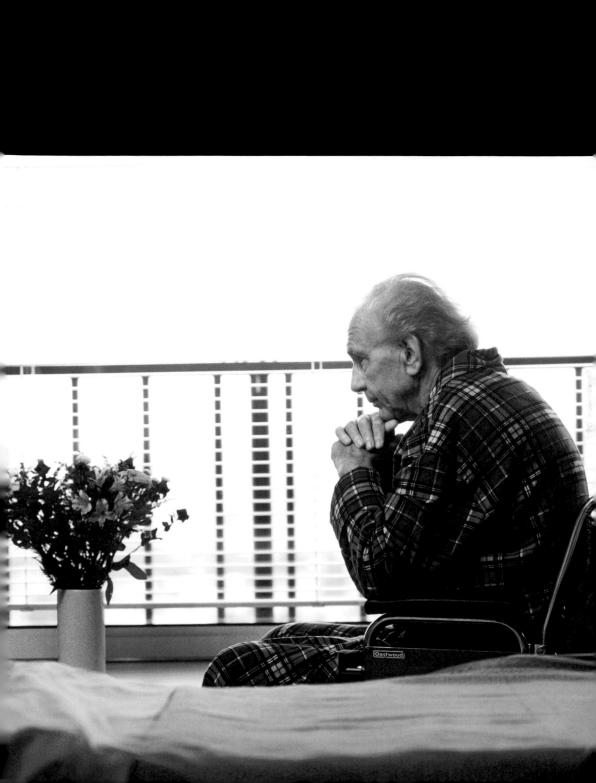

4

Science and Meditation

THE AUTONOMIC NERVOUS SYSTEM

THERE ARE TWO MAIN divisions of the body's nervous system. One division is voluntary (that is, it involves the will), and supplies impulses from the nerves to the voluntary muscles of the body like the arm or leg muscles. The other division is automatic, or "autonomic," supplying impulses from the nerves to the involuntary muscles throughout the body and the skin. These involuntary muscles are in many of the body's structures including the bowel wall, the walls of the blood vessels, and the heart. The autonomic nervous system also helps regulate the endocrine glands and the respiratory, circulatory, digestive, urinary, and genital systems. The name "autonomic nervous system" implies that these functions are automatic in most people. However, it is possible to learn to control either system while in meditation. When beginning, meditators learn to relax. They thereby lower blood pressure, decrease the pulse, and slow their respiration. Advanced yogic meditators have been reported to be able to stop the heart and suspend respiration for limited periods.

There are two divisions of the autonomic nervous system, and these are the sympathetic and the parasympathetic systems. They have opposite effects on the body. The first governs the "fight-or-flight" response, while the second has to do with the relaxation response.

The sympathetic system is activated by the body whenever there is a perceived threat, either physical or mental. The fight-or-flight response was very effective when humans were living in the wild and animals would physically attack people. Now, in our modern life, the fight-or-flight response is most often activated when there is a mental stress. This stress triggers the sympathetic nervous system to act directly on the body and also to release adrenalin. This causes constriction of the smooth muscles in the arteries of the extremities, which shuts off blood flow to the hands and feet—which then get cold. Cold hands are a common complaint among those who are feeling stressed. The constriction of the blood vessels will then cause an elevation of blood pressure. While the blood pressure goes up and the heart beats faster, there is more blood available for the brain and the muscles either to fight or to take flight. Unfortunately, prolonged high blood pressure causes damage to blood vessels and the heart. Reducing blood pressure to normal range is very important.

At the same time as the sympathetic nervous system is activated, a response along the hypothalamic-pituitary-adrenal axis is triggered. That is, the hypothalamic part of the brain signals the pituitary gland, at the base of the brain, to release a hormone that will stimulate the adrenal glands (which are next to the kidneys), to release cortisol from the cortex of the adrenal glands. Cortisol will cause elevation of blood sugar and depression of the immune system. All of these events combine to help the person be ready to fight or take flight.

This fight-or-flight reflex works well for us, but should only stay active for a short time. If the response persists for a long time (as we see happening a great deal in modern life) the body becomes "stressed out" and many diseases can develop. Much of the medicine prescribed today is to counter the effects of an overactive sympathetic nervous system. Yet meditation is very effective in countering the effects of the sympathetic nervous system without side effects and without great cost.

The opposite of the sympathetic nervous system is the parasympathetic nervous system, which can activate the relaxation response. Then, the heart is slowed, the hands become warm, blood pressure drops, digestion is stimulated, the person feels relaxed, and the cortisol level drops. This combination will slow down or even reverse the effects of stress. The immune system begins to function better and this will help the patient to heal. Breathing slows and the mind becomes calmer. Some feel more creative in this state. Activating the parasympathetic nervous system at will, with meditation as the tool, is a valuable skill in our stressful world.

STRESS

Stress was first described in the British journal *Nature* in the summer of 1936, by Hans Selye, M.D. He first described the General Adaptation Syndrome (GAS). This is the body's way of adapting to stress. Selye first observed stress in laboratory animals. He found that when stressed, the sympathetic nervous system is triggered and the body is ready to fight or take flight. This can energize the person to respond to the stressor.

Eustress is good stress; that is, stress that activates the sympathetic nervous system and gives us our competitive edge in performance-related activities like work, athletics, giving a speech, or acting, but it is short-acting and controlled. The body quickly returns from the higher sympathetic level to a lower, more normal level of sympathetic activation without the damaging effects of stress.

In chronic stress, the body adapts by keeping the sympathetic nervous system on continuous high alert. This is the stress that is common today with our fast pace of life. If there are additional stressors the body will not be able to react, as it is already overstimulated. This is the end stage, the unwelcome sort of stress that can eventually lead to collapse. It can lead to diseases common in the twenty-first century such as high blood pressure, indigestion, rapid heartbeat, cold hands, and tense muscles. It can also lead to asthma, irritable bowel syndrome, ulcers, headaches, back pain, skin disorders, coronary heart disease, psychological disorders such as depression and anxiety, and some cancers.

People also like to stress themselves artificially and stimulate the sympathetic nervous system to release adrenalin, which will cause a feeling of being "high." When high, the mind at first seems to work better and memory is improved. This high causes you to feel confident and helps you to get through the day. It causes you to feel stronger, mentally alert, less fearful, and able to work harder. The body initially engineered this adrenalin release as a lifesaver, but many are now using the adrenalin release to get their daily high. They have become "adrenalin junkies." For example, they schedule meetings too close together, not allowing enough time in between. Shortage of time is stressful and will trigger the fight-or-flight response, and then raise the body's adrenalin level. In many ways, throughout the day we consciously or unconsciously do things that will be stressful, raise adrenalin levels, and produce a high.

Humans also like to get their highs with stimulants like caffeine, medications, or illegal drugs. It is interesting that one of the most-consumed beverages around the world is coffee. This coffee consumption, combined with consumption of other caffeinated drinks, adds up to significant stimulant consumption. Illegal drugs, including cocaine and methamphetamine, also are used to create a high. Getting high is simply stressing the body and leads to many of the chronic diseases that are difficult and expensive to treat today.

There is a different high that can come from meditation. It is not a stimulated high from the sympathetic nervous system but a relaxed high that comes from triggering the parasympathetic system, one that allows the brain to focus and think on the task at hand. This ability to concentrate is called "being in the flow." When we are relaxed and in the flow, intuition and creativity are more available for use. Thinking is not as chaotic and scattered.

One of the challenges when learning to meditate comes from the part of the mind that likes to be stimulated and doesn't want to slow down. One of the values of meditation is that we can learn to calm this overstimulated mind, relax the body, and reduce the effects of stress.

SCIENCE AND STRESS

There are a number of scientific articles on the effects of stress, the most significant of which are reviewed below (for full references, see the list at the end). People who are regularly stressed show delayed immune response to vaccines, delayed wound healing, shortened life span, and altered autoimmunity diseases.

An excellent example of the effects of stress is described in an article in the journal *Scientific American*. Robert Sapolsky[15] discusses the effects of stress from poverty and how this stress causes disease and reduces life expectancy.

15   Sapolsky, 2005, 92-9.

He looks at the increase in disease and subsequent shortened life span among the poor and those on the lower rungs of society. The incidence of some diseases is tenfold higher for people in the lower rungs of the socio-economic ladder than on the upper rungs. Sapolsky is able to show that this effect of stress on the health of the poor and underprivileged is present even after subtracting the effects of poor sanitation, less medical care, and increased smoking, drug addiction, and other harmful factors. Living life in poverty on the lower rungs of society is very stressful and disease-producing.

He also describes a two-times higher death rate from heart disease in low-ranking British civil servants compared to the death rate of the higher-ranked administrators. Apparently, the rank and file are under more of the long-term stress that causes heart disease than their superiors. This doubled death rate also remains after allowance for other risk factors. His article adds to the research proving that stress can cause disease and is detrimental to long life. Finding ways to combat stress is important for everyone, most particularly the poor and those on the lower rungs of society.

PSYCHONEUROIMMUNOLOGY: THE STUDY OF HOW THE BRAIN IS CONNECTED TO THE IMMUNE SYSTEM

The immune system is connected to the nerves and then to the brain. The scientific proof for this connection between the brain and the immune system is being developed now. The scientific discipline that is concerned with studying this connection is called the field of Psychoneuroimmunology. PNI studies the central nervous system, the endocrine system, and the immune system. All of these parts of the body appear to be interconnected, thus explaining how thoughts can affect the immune system. Thoughts will affect the nerves, the hormones, and then the immune system, leading either to increased resistance or susceptibility to disease. Stress, as the studies show, has a noticeably deleterious effect on the immune system.

For instance, there is an excellent review of the field of PNI by Dr. Ronald Glaser,[16] who is a researcher at Ohio State University Medical Center. He has done extensive research on PNI. There is one study on medical students who were stressed by their studies. They became even more stressed when taking examinations. Glaser reports that "they studied academic stress, loneliness (as a modifier), stressful life events and their impact on urinary cortisol levels, NK cell activity (natural killer cells related to immunity), and the response of peripheral blood leukocytes (immune cells) to phytohemagglutinin as a measure of cellular immunity. Once again, a relationship was found with stress and these markers. Students who scored above the median on loneliness had significantly higher urinary cortisol levels and lowered response of their immune cells."[17]

---

16   Glaser, 2005, 3-11.

17   Kiecolt-Glaser et al., 1984.

In other studies, Glaser found that the immune response to vaccination was less in older individuals, medical students, and caregivers for Alzheimer's patients who were chronically stressed. His team proved this with flu and Hepatitis-B vaccines. They showed that the immune response was reduced and slower to take effect in those who were stressed. "The common thread through these viral vaccine studies is that immune dysregulation associated with psychological stressors can down-regulate both virus-specific antibody responses and, importantly, T-cell responses to antigens."

There is another excellent review of stress and immunology by Glaser and another researcher, D. A. Padgett, which shows the connection between the brain and the rest of the body.[18] Padgett and Glaser say "stress diminishes vaccine responses, exacerbates viral and bacterial pathogenesis, slows wound healing and alters autoimmune diseases (such as rheumatoid arthritis and Crohn's disease)." They show the effects of stress are extensive, particularly with chronic, hard-to-treat diseases. It is estimated that "more than 60 percent of visits to physicians in the United States are due to stress-related problems, many of which are poorly treated by drugs, surgery or other medical procedures."[19]

---

18   Padgett and Glaser, 2003.

19   Herbert Benson, M.D., in Cromie, 2002, 2.

The crucial importance of meditation is that it can reduce the effects of stress. This in part explains why it can be effective in the treatment of chronic disease.

Glaser also reports[20] that wound healing can be influenced by stress. There have been a number of controlled studies where a small punch biopsy wound or a blister was created and then the rate of healing of this wound was measured. There was a definite delay in wound healing in those who were stressed. Caregivers of dementia patients, a traditionally highly stressed group, had a 24 percent delay in wound healing in one study. Another study of wound healing after surgery found that healing was delayed by at least one day if the patient was stressed just before surgery. [21]

Another researcher, Candace Pert, has done extensive research in the fields of psychoneuroimmunology and psychoneuropharmacology. She has worked on peptides (small proteins) that affect the body. She feels that there is a feedback system linking the brain and the body, using peptide molecules. The brain and then the body are affected by our thoughts and emotions. Well-known on both sides of the Atlantic for her work, she has lectured extensively

---

20 Glaser, 2005, 7.

21 Kiecolt-Glaser et al., 2005, 62.

and has been featured in the United States with Bill Moyers on the PBS series *Healing and the Mind.*[22]

It is becoming obvious that understanding and controlling stress in our lives is important. Chronic stress is all too common today among the electronic generation. It has been estimated that those who live in the United States are at least one hour short of sleep every day. Add this to a day filled with emails, mobile phones, and automobile traffic, and there is a recipe for chronic stress. If this goes on too long, you can enter the final phase Hans Selye described, the one of exhaustion. When exhausted, the body is not able to function well, and that allows physical and mental diseases to really take hold. Regular meditation is great as an antidote because it is a tool that we can use to control or reduce the effects of stress, to break up chronic stress, and thus to improve our health.

RESULTS OF RESEARCH ON MEDITATION

Science is investigating the underlying effects of meditation, effects that are common to everyone. Humans are similar, with similar bodies and minds. No matter which meditation technique is used, the mind and body can only react in certain ways. Research is finding that there is much in common between the schools of meditation. In the past, the only knowledge of meditation came from reports of experienced meditators or from personal anecdotes. These re-

---

22   For a review of her work, see Neimark, 1997.

ports were often difficult to interpret. Now, new scientific techniques are being used to study the effects of meditation. Part of the mystery of meditation is being replaced by knowledge gained from scientific study. These research procedures are also used on patients under hypnosis, which is another altered state with some similarities to meditation. Although hypnosis and meditation are similar we shall see there are differences between them.[23] We are beginning to learn about the different parts of the brain involved in meditation and other altered states, and what their function is. With the new PET, fMRI, CT, and SPECT scanners, as well as EEGs (a technology which will be described shortly), we can correlate different anatomic areas of the brain with observations made in meditation and hypnosis.

It is well to caution, however, that in the initial period of meditation research there was enthusiastic reporting about the effects of meditation by some authors. Some of these claims have not proven to be correct when closely examined. Fortunately, double-blinded studies, which use a normal control group for comparison with the treatment group, are becoming common. In addition, the new scanning machines, which are very accurate, make a whole new level of analysis possible.

There are now thousands of scientific research articles on meditation. We have already mentioned some of the leading names in the field, such as Herbert Benson, Ronald Glaser, and Candace Pert; other important researchers

---

23   See p. 34.

include Jon Kabat-Zinn, Ph.D.; Dean Ornish, M.D.; Deepak Chopra, M.D.; Andrew Weil, M.D.; Esther M. Sternberg, M.D.; and the researchers at the Transcendental Meditation University. There are many others who have written and spoken extensively about the effects of meditation and how meditation can influence your health.

There is an excellent book by Michael Murphy and Steven Donovan called *The Physical and Psychological Effects of Meditation* that comprehensively reviews much of the past research on meditation. This work originates from a nonprofit group, the Institute of Noetic Sciences (www.noetic.org), which has compiled a large library of research on meditation.

A discussion of the effects of meditation requires an understanding of the meaning of the words used by its different schools. For research results to be understandable and reproducible, a common language is necessary. This standardized meditation language is being developed as there is sharing of information by researchers and meditation teachers from around the world.

In the early days of research into meditation, easily measured physiological parameters of the autonomic nervous system such as pulse and respiration were examined. When equipment to measure blood pressure and the galvanic response of the skin became available, more effects of meditation were documented. Then it became possible to study additional effects of the autonomic nervous system by doing laboratory tests on the blood, checking hormone, peptide, and white blood-cell levels.

Now, those doing research are able to observe the brain's anatomy as it is functioning. New scanning machines make this possible. Electroencephalography (EEG), Positive Emission Tomography (PET), Single Photon Emission Commuted Tomography (SPECT), Computed Tomography (CT), and functional Magnetic Resonance Imaging (fMRI) machines are available, allowing researchers to look at brain anatomy and brain blood flow, real-time. It is currently possible to compare the experiences reported by meditators with their simultaneously obtained brain scans. In other words, researchers can observe what happens to the brain while you are thinking or meditating. These machines will tell which part of the brain is activated during different mental or meditative activities.

EEG testing is done by putting electrodes on the surface of the head. These electrodes pick up the electrical activity of the brain. The electrical activity changes with different types of brain function such as sleep or mental calculations. The brainwaves from the area of the brain that is active will be recorded on the EEG. There are four different brainwave types: alpha, beta, delta, and theta. Beta waves are used when the brain is aroused and highly active. Alpha waves are the major rhythms seen in normal, relaxed adults, and can be increased by deep breathing. Delta waves come with deep sleep. Among the times that theta waves are noted are the meditative state and when the person is "in the flow." Researchers use EEG recordings to determine when a person is in a meditative state.

PET scans are done with a radioactive isotope that is injected into the blood. The radiation dose is very small and not harmful. The isotope is a safe molecule that is made to go to a specific part of the body such as the brain, heart, or liver. PET scans will show where in the brain there is hypermetabolic activity. The isotope will go to the part of the body where there is increased glucose metabolism; in other words, the part of the brain that is very active at that time. With PET scans, we can then localize the part of the brain activated by certain types of meditation. This information is correlated with the experiences reported by the meditator and the EEG of the meditator to give hard scientific evidence about the effects of meditation on the brain.

MRI (magnetic resonance imaging) is a new technique used to image the brain. The MRI machine works using magnetism. The patient is placed in a large magnet and the tests are done. It is nice to note the tests have been proven to be safe. The MRI machines are widely used in medicine as they give very detailed anatomic pictures of the brain and nervous system. MRI scans give detailed pictures of the brain, but the images are static and only show the static anatomy of the brain. By contrast, fMRI (functional MRI) gives ongoing pictures while the brain is functioning. It is very useful in mapping the brain while people are meditating. With this type of scan it is possible to detect the changes that are ongoing during meditation. With the new techniques for testing we are beginning to have real, scientific, and reproducible findings about meditation.

You can also measure the immune system by testing the blood level of different types of white blood cells (NK and T cells) and blood proteins such as peptides (small proteins). Your thoughts can affect the immune system, as has been proven and is discussed later, in the section on the results of scientific research into meditation. You can affect the immune system by meditating in ways that can lead to improved health.

What follows is an overview of what is known scientifically about meditation and its effects on the body.

HEART RATE

Generally the heart rate slows in meditation as the person quiets down and activates the relaxation response. The heart rate slowing can be varied, but it is usually in the range of seven to ten beats per minute. Long-time meditators can lower their heart rates more. As I mentioned earlier, advanced yogis have reputedly been able to stop their hearts for short periods. There can also be a more permanent lowering of heart rate with long-term meditation. There is an unusual subset of advanced meditators who experience an elevation of pulse with some special forms of meditation, such as one called "breath of fire," but in general the pulse slows with meditation.[24]

BLOOD PRESSURE (BP)

Many experiments indicate that blood pressure drops when the relaxation response is triggered. The range of BP reduction varies, but there can be five to twenty millimeters of mercury reduction in BP. This means that the upper (systolic) and lower (diastolic) numbers decrease. The lowering effect will persist if the person continues meditation practice. Meditation can be included in the medical treatment of hypertension. It can be used alone or as a supplement to medication. When used as a supplement, it will allow a lower dose of the BP medicine, which will reduce the side effects of the medication.

BLOOD FLOW

There is increased blood flow to the brain during meditation. The frontal lobes gain a larger blood flow.

BRAINWAVE TYPES

There have been many experiments using EEGs to record the results of meditation on meditators. The EEGs show a change in meditators' brainwaves when compared with those of non-meditators. Meditation creates different

---

24   Peng et al., 1995.

brainwaves, as measured by EEG. "Evidence that meditation leads to an increase in alpha rhythms is extensive.... A characteristic brainwave pattern of long-term meditators includes strong bursts of frontally dominant theta rhythms, during which meditators report peaceful, drifting, and generally pleasant experiences with intact self-awareness."[25] These tests have been done on advanced Indian yogis as well as Western meditators. The EEG results are compatible with the findings that are coming from testing with the newer MRI and PET scanners.

CORTISOL AND ADRENALIN

The adrenal gland has an outer cortex that releases cortisol and an inner medulla that releases adrenalin. These are two very important hormones that are related to stress and can be related to disease.

Cortisol lowers immune function, raises blood pressure, and raises blood-sugar levels. With chronic stress, high cortisol levels can be damaging to the body. Cortisol levels fall with meditation.

Adrenalin is the hormone that is produced when there is stress and stimulation of the sympathetic nervous system as described above. Adrenalin levels will lower for some who meditate.

---

25   Murphy and Donovan, 57.

CHOLESTEROL

This blood product produced by the liver during stress has been shown to decrease with meditation, with decreases up to 25 mg/dl (milligrams/deciliter) in those who meditate regularly. The normal level should be lower than 200 mg/dl to help prevent heart and blood vessel disease. Meditation can lower the cholesterol level as much as some medication can. This reduction in cholesterol with the practice of meditation is likely due to reduction in sympathetic nervous system activity.

OXYGEN CONSUMPTION AND MUSCLE TENSION

Both of these are lowered with meditation. The body's metabolism (the chemical reactions in the body that produce energy and consume oxygen) is lowered, reducing the demands on the body.

CORTICAL THICKENING OF THE BRAIN

New research using an MRI scanner was completed by Lazar and others on twenty participants with extensive insight-meditation experience. The researchers discovered that parts of the brain grew thicker with meditation. This is a significant finding offering the hope that meditation could help prevent the loss of brain tissue that usually comes with aging. It may even be possible to regain some of the brain tissue that was lost previously. "Brain regions associated with attention and sensory processing were thicker in meditation participants than matched controls, including the prefrontal cortex and right anterior insula. Between-group differences in prefrontal cortical thickness were most pronounced in older participants, suggesting that meditation might offset age-related cortical thinning. Finally, the thickness of the two regions correlated with meditation experience."[26]

FRONTAL LOBE AND BASAL GANGLIA PARTS OF THE BRAIN

More research using MRI or PET scanning is being reported on the effects of meditation on the brain. A group in Denmark studied eleven experienced Zen meditation practitioners using fMRI. There was increased "activity of the prefrontal cortex (gyrus frontalis medius, right side, Brodmann area) during Zen meditation…. The gyrus frontalis medius is part of the frontal lobe…. Also the basal ganglia became more active during the meditation periods in our study."[27]

Research using SPECT scans of eight meditators found frontal lobe enhancement during meditation.[28] There was also an increase in thalamic activity in the basal ganglia. The researchers also reported that the changes they had seen in the frontal and parietal cortices during the meditation session were closely related to the positive mental states that are described during meditation.

---

26   Lazar et al., 2005, 1893-7.

27   Ritskes et al., 2002.

28   Newberg et al., 2001.

These articles describe increased activity in the frontal areas and basal ganglia during meditation. Such findings prove that meditation has a physical effect as well as a psychological or spiritual one, which can be correlated with positive mental states. Meditation is not some fake made-up event, but it has measurable effects.

PRODUCTION OF DOPAMINE

Dopamine is a neurotransmitter, a brain chemical that transmits impulses from nerve to nerve. It is necessary for some nerves to function. Researchers used a PET scanner to measure dopamine release in the brain during meditation. They correlated PET scan results with the reports of subjects using a deep meditative practice known as *yoga nidra*. They were "characterized by a depressed level of desire for action, associated with decreased blood flow in the prefrontal, cerebellar and subcortical regions." Two scans were done, one while the meditators were speaking and one while they were meditating. They found that there was a 65 percent increase in endogenous (internal in the brain) dopamine release during meditation. Not only did they have the reports of the meditators, they had additional correlation from EEG measurements. There were theta waves, a characteristic feature of meditation on the EEG. They showed increased striatal dopamine release during meditation. They concluded that they had demonstrated *in vivo* (that is, by a test in a living organism) evidence for regulation of conscious states at a synaptic level (the level in the brain where nerve junctions meet).[29] In other words, what we think consciously has an effect physically on the brain.

EEG MEASUREMENT AND IMMUNE RESPONSE

Another team of researchers "measured electrical brain activity … and found significant increases in left-sided anterior activation, a pattern previously associated with positive effect, in the meditators compared with non-meditators." They also measured the response to the influenza vaccine and found that the meditators had a stronger immune response to the influenza vaccine. Importantly they found that the stronger meditators, as measured by EEG, had a stronger immune response. "The magnitude of increase in left-sided activation (on EEG) predicted the magnitude of antibody-level rise to the vaccine." They concluded, "Meditation may change brain and immune function in positive ways."[30]

Regarding the opening of atherosclerotic blood vessels: There have been studies suggesting that meditation has a beneficial effect on blood vessels. The original work was done by Dean Ornish, M.D.,[31] who found that coronary arteries in the heart would open up without medication. He used a program of meditation, low-fat diet, and yoga. His work was revolutionary. Doctors

---

29   Kjaer et al., 2002.

30   Davidson et al., 2001.

31   *Dr. Dean Ornish's Program for Reversing Heart Disease.*

at that time assumed that arteries which were narrowed by plaques (atherosclerosis) could not be opened without surgery or balloon angioplasty. To establish a baseline for the study, he did angiography on the coronary blood vessels of the heart to determine the size of the opening of the arteries at the beginning of the experiment. He then put the patients on his treatment regimen for one year and did a repeat angiogram, which demonstrated that the coronary arteries had opened up. The plaque in the arteries had decreased. His work has been duplicated in many centers around the world. Later work demonstrated that there was more plaque regression with a five-year treatment regimen.[32]

There is some question about how much meditation contributed to the results as Ornish also included a low-fat diet, counseling, and yoga with his treatment. A new study by Amparo Castillo-Richmond, M.D. and others[33] suggests that blood vessels will open with meditation only. There were sixty men and women in the study. They did Transcendental Meditation twice daily for six to nine months. At the end of the study, the carotid arteries showed opening with a reduction of atherosclerosis. The opening was minimal, but Castillo-Richmond thought it was significant. They also had a reduction in blood pressure and heart rate which may have helped the arteries. They did their measurements on the carotid arteries (arteries to the brain)

---

32 Ornish et al., 1998.

33 Castillo-Richmond et al., 2000.

using B-mode ultrasound. More work needs to be done in this area with studies done over a longer time.

There appear to be many factors that will reduce the amount of atherosclerosis in patients' arteries. These include diet, meditation, yoga, and counseling. Until more data is available it is best to do the combined program recommended by Ornish: low-fat diet, exercise, meditation, counseling, and yoga. The Ornish program has been proven over a number of years.

SKIN DISEASE

Jon Kabat-Zinn, a leading researcher, and others "reported that mindful meditation-based stress reduction intervention delivered by audiotape during ultraviolet light therapy can increase the rate of resolution of psoriatic lesions in patients with psoriasis." Healing of the skin disease psoriasis was helped by practicing simple meditation techniques given on an audiotape.[34]

ANXIETY

There are many studies showing the effect of meditation on the mind. There are excellent studies showing good results with anxious patients. Another team "showed that medical patients with anxiety disorders showed clinically and statistically significant improvements in subjective and objective symp-

---

34   Kabat-Zinn et al., 1998.

toms of anxiety and panic."[35] This reduced-anxiety effect was shown to continue through three months and then three years.

MEDITATION AND PSYCHOTHERAPY

In a review by *US Newswire*, the April 2005 issue of the *Harvard Mental Health Letter* was said to have reported that "meditation is now being incorporated into psychotherapeutic practice and combined in surprising ways with other healing traditions.... The psychotherapeutic tradition now taking meditation most seriously is cognitive behavioral therapy ... merging cognitive techniques and meditation in something they call the 'third wave' of cognitive behavioral therapy, called mindfulness-based cognitive therapy."[36] Psychologists are combining psychological talk therapy with meditation to achieve good results.

ORGAN TRANSPLANT PATIENTS

C. R. Gross and others studied the effects of mindfulness meditation on patients who had received solid-organ (heart, lung, kidney, pancreas, and liver) transplants. They evaluated depression, anxiety, sleep disturbance, and quality of life after solid-organ transplantation. At three months there was improvement in sleep and anxiety levels directly related to the time spent meditating.

---

35   Miller et al., 1995.

36   *US Newswire*, April 20, 2005.

Depression scores were no different from the baseline. They suggested further trials as patients in the study demonstrated improvement.[37]

CANCER AND MEDITATION

A randomized controlled study has been done of ninety patients with various types and stages of cancer who meditated for seven weeks in a ninety-minute weekly class and also did home meditation. Those who meditated had a reduction of 65 percent in mood disturbance (depression, anxiety, anger, and confusion) and a 31 percent reduction in the symptoms of stress. Researchers confirmed the positive effects of meditation.[38]

There is ongoing work by multiple researchers on the effects of meditation and cancer treatment. Their preliminary results show a reduction in stress hormones and an improvement in the quality of life. There are additional early findings that a reduction in stress will strengthen the immune system and help with healing of HIV and cancer. Visualization of the immune system killing cancer cells is postulated by some to be helpful with cancer. This effect has not been definitely proven at this time.

---

37   Gross, 2004.

38   Specca et al., 2000.

CHRONIC PAIN

Jon Kabat-Zinn reports on the reduction of chronic pain with meditation. He states, "Statistically significant reductions were observed in measures of present-moment pain, negative body image, inhibition of activity by pain, symptoms, mood disturbance, and psychological symptomatology, including anxiety and depression. Pain-related drug utilization decreased and activity levels and feelings of self-esteem increased."[39]

CONTROL OF BODY TEMPERATURE

With more meditation experience, the meditator has greater control over the body. Meditators can learn to slow the heart rate and change body temperature. Tibetan monks can raise their body temperature enough to dry out a wet sheet placed over their shoulders in temperatures of 49° F (9.5°C).

Research is showing there are practical benefits of meditation, including control of body heat to aid in survival, improved healing, lowered blood pressure, lowered pain, and improvement against chronic diseases.

SCIENCE AND THE BRAIN

There has been considerable research on the brain. The terminology used to describe the brain and the mind is confusing. For this book I will talk about

---

39   Kabat-Zinn et al., 1985.

the part of the brain that is active during everyday living, and the part of the brain that is little used daily, but can be active during meditation and hypnosis. To distinguish, I shall sometimes refer to this part as the "higher levels," but in the sense of more remote from the everyday, not a different geographical situation. When the mind is accessed during meditation and hypnosis there are changes in the brain that can be measured scientifically.

"Hypnosis is a sleep-like state usually induced by another person in which forgotten or suppressed memories, hallucinations, and heightened suggestibility may be experienced."[40] There are hundreds of articles and books on hypnosis. It has been used widely. Hypnosis has been used effectively in many areas including smoking cessation, pain reduction, and psychotherapy. After relaxation, which is common to both hypnosis and meditation, both techniques access the higher mind. With hypnosis, there are goals and hoped-for results that are suggested by the therapist. With meditation we are free to explore and experience the higher mind as we wish. We can watch our mind unfold and be aware of our thoughts.

New research on hypnosis was reported in *The New York Times* in November 2005. The research was done with fMRI brain imaging. It showed that it is possible to change perception of visual stimuli.[41] Normally, sensory information

---

40 *American Heritage College Dictionary.*

41 *The New York Times*, November 11, 2005.

enters the nervous system and then is sent to the mind to be processed and interpreted. This is a "bottom-up" system.

This research, however, shows that perception of your sensations is actually controlled by the mind. The mind can override and reinterpret the input coming up from the sensory nervous system. This is a "top-down" system that reinterprets sensations. What we see, hear, feel, and believe is based on what neuroscientists call "top-down processing." What you see is not always what you get. It may be what the mind wants you to think it is.

If this is true, then hypnosis works by the therapist suggesting an idea to the mind and suggesting a change in how you perceive your sensory inputs, such as pain. For example, during hypnosis most people who are instructed not to feel pain on the back of their hand will not feel pain when a needle is put through the skin of the back of their hand. They will not feel the needle. The patient's mind is ignoring the sensory input from the needle stick. This ability of the mind to override and reinterpret incoming sensations has large implications. If you can access the little-used part of the brain in hypnosis or meditation, you have the opportunity to work with the mind and body in positive ways. One of these ways, once regarded as an obstacle to scientific study but now seriously studied in its own right, is known as the placebo effect.

The placebo effect is described in the Encarta Dictionary as "a psychological effect of treatment, a sense of benefit felt by a patient that arises solely from the knowledge that treatment has been given." There is an excellent review of the placebo effect by Fabrizio Benedetti.[42] He reports on an improvement in patients with Parkinson's disease after the administration of a placebo. If the patient has high expectancy of improvement with a medication (placebo), there is an increase in endogenous dopamine released in the brain, demonstrated on a PET scan. This release of dopamine comes from the patient's own brain and is not caused by medication or anything from outside. The patient's Parkinson's symptoms will improve. This is an amazing finding, suggesting humans have the ability to improve themselves just by giving suggestions to the mind. It is possible to make disease better or worse with positive or negative thinking.

It has been shown with many studies that when the patient believes in a medication's effectiveness, even though it is only a sugar pill, the patient will improve around 40 percent of the time. The placebo effect is stronger if the patient has great expectancy that the medicine will work. The way that the placebo is administered will change the effect. If a doctor (or advertising) really sells the benefits of the medication, the placebo effect will be greater. The placebo effect will work because the higher levels of the mind interpret the placebo as an effective medication. It is becoming clearer that what the higher mind believes about a treatment will affect how you respond to that treatment. The brain has a way to affect the body without actual treatment given.

---

42   Benedetti et al., 2005.

Modern medicine is beginning to incorporate some of these findings into the treatment and care of patients.

Words are powerful in many ways. Words can have a positive or negative effect on the brain. Negative thoughts can be stressful and lead to depression of the immune system. Positive thoughts can strengthen the immune system. Positive or negative thinking can influence the PNI system. There is something to the "power of positive thinking," a phrase first coined as a book title as long ago as 1952. Words will affect how you feel about yourself. When a student is expected to do well and then be rewarded, the student will work hard and do well. If the student is the scapegoat and negatively rewarded, then he or she will not perform well.

Self-talk, when you talk to yourself either verbally or inside your mind, is powerful as well. If your self-talk is positive then you will feel better and more self-confident. You can use affirmations for positive self-talk. An affirmation has the words "I am" and then a positive statement. For example, the affirmation "I am happy" repeated over and over will help you to be happy. Other affirmations work very well such as "I am calm," "I am feeling good," and "I will do well today." It is amazing how often a positive attitude with positive self-talk will lead to success. Negative talk and thinking will lead to depression and failure. It then becomes obvious that it is important to be positive with yourself and other people.

Talk therapy or cognitive psychotherapy is very effective. The mind is capable of accepting suggestions, learning, and then changing. The therapist and the client work together to help the client have positive and constructive thoughts that can assist management of life.

The mind has been studied extensively in many ways. It is progressively being better understood. Meditation offers a way for you to learn about your mind whenever you so desire. You can learn who you are and then begin to change the thoughts that are limiting you. It is a wonderful tool to help you—one that is inexpensive and very effective.

SCIENCE AND THE RELAXATION RESPONSE

When the relaxation response is triggered, your muscles relax, your blood pressure drops, your heart-rate slows, and your immune system strengthens. In addition, your breathing will slow and the mind's attention will be on the object of your meditation.

This is the first stage of meditation. Most meditation techniques will help the meditator achieve relaxation. Prior to 1950, it was thought you had to meditate in a certain way, as taught by certain religions, to achieve this relaxation. Several religions use a mantra to achieve this relaxation. The mantra was a secret word, given by the teacher in the meditation class. It was repeated over and over again to begin meditation. This repetition caused a purely physical effect, the relaxation response, which by now we have mentioned several times, and is also common to most other types of meditation. Herbert Benson, who identified the response, wondered if a person could achieve this level of relaxation using a technique that was free of religion, and in doing so he made a major contribution. In his classic account of the response, he described the four basic elements to bring forth the relaxation response, namely a quiet environment, an object to dwell upon, a passive attitude, and a comfortable position.

He suggested that if the four elements above are in place, a simple way to trigger the relaxation response is simply to say a single word over and over again. Any word will suffice. The word becomes an object the mind can focus on, and then the mind can become calm, and the relaxation response will be initiated. Transcendental meditation, mindfulness meditation, and other types of meditation will all trigger the relaxation response. There are many other techniques that will also access the relaxation response including progressive relaxation, biofeedback, hypnosis, or praying a rosary.

THINGS TO REMEMBER:

1. There are many new scientific discoveries about meditation.

2. Meditation can trigger the relaxation response and reduce the negative effects of stress.

3. There are immediate and long-term beneficial physical changes that can occur with meditation.

4. Meditation is effective in the treatment of some diseases, particularly chronic, hard-to-treat ones.

5. Meditation is being combined with psychotherapy with good results.

6. There is a connection between the central nervous system, the endocrine glands, and the immune system. Meditation can access this system and help improve immunity and healing.

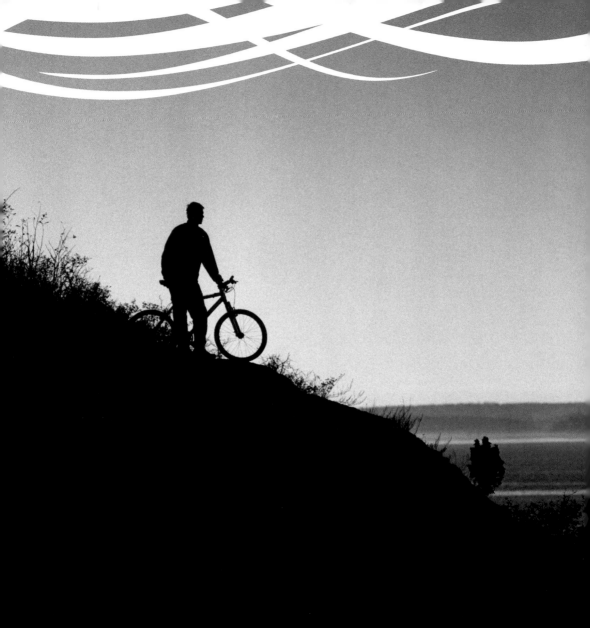

5

Meditation

THE BEST WAY TO MEDITATE

THE QUESTION COMES UP FREQUENTLY: what is the best way to meditate? The answer is any way that you will follow regularly. All types of meditation have some value. Simply learning how to relax and lower stress will improve health. Deeper understanding of the mind will free us of some of the anxieties and fears that are causing difficulties in daily living. Spiritual closeness and an awareness of a higher place give us peace and take away some of the fear of death. All of these things are good.

One of the early challenges in learning to meditate is finding the right school of meditation for you. Meditation can be learned with or without religious overtones. As we know, the relaxation response can be initiated with the simple repetition of a word. This can be done in a class or at home quite effectively. A class will offer structure and support that is very helpful. There are also many books on meditation with or without religious teachings that are quite effective. Cassettes, CDs, and DVDs are also widely available. In all of this, personal recommendation is likely to be the greatest help.

Many people in the West are learning a path of meditation that combine teachings from both the East and the West and can be non-religious or religious. Once a path of meditation is chosen, it is best to stick with it for a while rather than jumping around from one to another.

HOW DO I START MEDITATING?

Learning to meditate alone using a book or an audio device is quite possible, and this book and CD will get you started; however, it is easier to learn if you attend a meditation class. It is up to you to research the best type of class for you. It is also good to read several other books on meditation to get a sample of the different types of meditation available. This book contains a bibliography that lists several other meditation books.

Before choosing a type of meditation, the following are some of the questions that need to be answered.

1. What types of meditation classes are available in your area?

2. Do you want a meditation class with religious teachings or without? If the former, what are the religious teachings? Are you comfortable with them?

3. Do you want to be able to choose which type of focus to use for meditating? Many Eastern and some Western traditions use a mantra, the repetition of a word, to begin meditation. Other

groups use visualization of an image. Others use the breath, and some the observation of our thoughts. The types of meditation are different, each with its own advantages.

4. Do you want to meditate sitting down or does movement meditation sound better? If you prefer to be seated, does the class give you the option of being cross-legged on the floor or seated on a chair?

5. Movement meditation classes are widely available. In yoga, tai chi, or qi gong classes, teachers will give you various movements or poses that become meditative with practice. Although I class it as a movement meditation, hatha yoga has mostly static poses while tai chi and qi gong have flowing movements. Yoga, tai chi, or qi gong methods are all valuable. It is best not to mix them up at first, so try one and stay with it for a series of classes until you have a basic understanding of the concept behind the teachings.

If you have time during the years ahead, try several different meditation methods to find out which one you like the best. Many people do both sitting and movement meditation with excellent results.

It is best not to combine illegal drugs and meditation. In the past there was experimentation with illegal drugs, like LSD, to enhance the meditative experience. Many report an "experience," sometimes spiritual, when they take drugs. Unfortunately, illegal drugs can cause permanent alteration to the brain. Mental illness may develop. The drugs can be addictive. It is possible not to return to normal functioning from a drug "trip." It is strongly advised not to take illegal drugs. Meditation has the advantage of being free, non-toxic, and non-addictive.

MEDITATION FOR RELAXATION

It is perfectly possible to begin meditating on your own. The following is a checklist of things you need to begin a successful meditation practice.

1. A commitment to meditate regularly.
2. A quiet room without distractions like telephones.
3. A comfortable sitting position.
4. A chosen focus for your attention. This could be mindfulness of your breath, a repeated word, or visualization of an image of beauty.
5. Comfortable clothes—these are a must.
6. A clear mind, with no alcohol, illegal drugs, or caffeine.
7. A happy stomach—not empty or stuffed.

Focusing the mind is the big challenge for you as a novice. The mind is used to running your life, and in meditation it wants to continue to be boss. Your challenge is to switch your mind's attention from distracting ideas to being mindful of an object, word, or image.

MINDFULNESS

Mindfulness is the observation and heightened awareness of an object. To be mindful of something you look at it, become aware of it, think about it, and are receptive to what you are seeing. As your mind focuses on the object, let all of your distracting thoughts drift away. As a distracting thought comes into your mind, it is important to let the distracting idea go and bring the attention of your mind back to mindful observation of a word, object, or image. As you begin to concentrate and focus, you will begin to meditate. With practice, you will feel an internal shift as you access the relaxation response.

The following things can be used as a focus for meditation.

1. A word

Simply repeat a word or mantra over and over again. When a stray idea comes into your mind, bring your attention back to the word. After time the mind settles down and relaxation begins. At first it may be necessary to return to the word many times to get your mind settled down. Everyone has distracting thoughts when meditating.

The important thing is to keep bringing your mind back to the word or other focal point. This is the technique used by Herbert Benson in the "relaxation response," and it also is the technique used by many other meditation traditions.

2.   The breath

After closing your eyes to the outer world, breathe out, and now let yourself take a deep breath. Observe and feel your breath as it passes into the lungs. What does the breath feel like as it goes through your nose and down into the lungs? What do the muscles feel like, expanding and contracting with each breath? If a distracting idea comes into your mind, let it go and bring your mind's attention back to the breath. Carry on watching the breath, without any effort, just using the rhythm that comes naturally. This is a very simple but very effective technique. This technique has also been used in medicine, particularly in childbirth, to reduce the awareness of pain.

3.   An object

Focus your attention on a physical object and be mindful of how it looks. Jon Kabat-Zinn[43] has his students be mindful of a raisin. His students observe, smell, feel and finally taste the raisin. This in its totality is what being mindful of a raisin means. You can be mindful

---

43   *Full Catastrophe Living: Using the Wisdom of Your Body and Mind to Face Stress, Pain, and Illness.*

of a flower or a less static object like a flame. The mind can become occupied with mindful observation of this object, diverting attention from distracting thoughts. When a distracting thought comes into your mind, bring your attention back to the object you have chosen.

4. The sensation of movement

After taking a class in yoga, tai chi or qi gong, you can practice at home. With time you will begin to experience a form of meditation as you practice the movements. Yoga, tai chi or qi gong will help you with your sitting meditation and will also help you maintain flexibility.

Note that movement and sitting meditations are equally good. You will notice additional benefits to your life by practicing both movement meditation and sitting meditation. You can first do yoga, tai chi or qi gong movements and then do a sitting meditation. The yoga postures were designed to quiet the body for meditation. The combination of both types of meditation is widely practiced around the world.

5. Visualization

With this method, you focus on an image formed in your inner mind. Examples of images include flowers, lakes, gardens, jewels, mountains, or other beautiful things you like. For many people this is an easy way to meditate. To begin with, in your mind visualize something beautiful. It helps to have an image that is familiar and meaningful to you. Observe the image with the inner eyes, outer eyes are closed. Look at the image in a mindful way and mentally describe it. The five senses can be used internally when observing an image in meditation.

As meditation deepens, your mindful attention will allow you to almost be as one with the image. For example, if a flower is the focus for the meditation, it is possible to imagine being the flower and feel rain or sun shining on your petals. Again, if there are distracting ideas that intrude, let them go and don't think about them. But rather than fighting them, simply bring your attention back to the visualization. With visualization meditation, your appreciation of beauty becomes greater. You can detect an improvement in your ability to sense the outer world. Colors become more vivid, smells are more subtle, and music is felt at a deeper level.

It is also possible for you to imagine yourself in the scene you are visualizing. You can walk along a path, perhaps in a garden, along a lake, or in a forest. It is possible for you to have animals or birds in your meditation if you wish. You are creating the image, so it can be as beautiful as you like.

You can also visualize the body in meditation. It is possible to visualize the breath moving through the nose. You visualize the breath going in one nostril and out the other, alternately. Whether you visualize this happening or do it by blocking a nostril with your finger, it will help balance the brain.

Relaxing meditation, as above, is great for starting the relaxation response and reducing the effects of stress. Stress is the cause of much disease. By learning how to relax whenever you desire, you can improve your health. You can bring your body back into balance and harmony.

MEDITATION ON THE MIND

During meditation on the mind, thoughts are examined and observed. To help you make this journey through the mind you have a part of your brain that is called the observer. In other words, you can observe your thoughts and actions as you act and interface with your friends and fellow travelers here on earth. You can observe a thought, name the thought, go on to the next thought, and with time detect the pattern of your thoughts. You can observe a personal trait and then examine the reasons that caused you to have this trait. You can look at the layers of your mind this way.

Though I am describing it in a simplified way, this is what insight or *vipassana* meditation is in the Buddhist and yogic tradition. There are many writings about what experienced insight meditation practitioners have found. Several particularly clear Buddhist writers include Joseph Goldstein, Jack Kornfield, the present Dalai Lama, and Thich Nhat Hanh. Stephan Bodian, who has a background in yoga, has also written clearly on this sort of meditation.[44] Their writings are very helpful with the understanding of meditation.

In the book *Seeking the Heart of Wisdom*, Joseph Goldstein and Jack Kornfield say, "When we stop struggling and let be, the natural wisdom, joy, and freedom of our being emerges and expresses itself effortlessly. Our actions can come out of spontaneous compassion and our innate wisdom can direct life from our heart. In meditation we learn to care with a full-hearted attention, true caring for each moment. Yet we also learn to let go. We do not separate out only those experiences we enjoy, but cultivate a sense of harmony, opening constantly to the truth within us and connecting with all life."[45]

SPIRITUAL MEDITATION

The spiritual realm is hard to describe, as it is unseen in the conventional sense. It is a very beautiful and interesting realm which has been described by spiritual teachers and aspirants from many faiths. It is a world that is not easily measured and examined, but can be explored in meditation, as millions have done over the ages. Some skeptics scoff at the idea of a spiritual world that cannot be seen with earthly eyes. However, in meditation you can have deeply moving spiritual experiences that may convince you there is a spiritual

---

44 *Meditation for Dummies*, 221-2.

45 p. 57.

world. Initially, you may use your creativity to "see" beautiful images; gradually, meditators say, they may become spontaneous.

Some people describe spiritual meditation as a communion with a higher being. Some have had experiences where they have received Christian communion while in the spiritual realm.

This spiritual world has numerous levels. Many traditional religions have a description of a beautiful "heaven" with spiritual beings and loved ones. These spiritual levels can be experienced with different techniques of meditation. Visualization meditation, as it has been discussed, is a very useful approach in spiritual meditation. The creative part of the mind that visualizes can be used as a door to the spiritual world.

Heaven is described as beautiful. Walks through gardens or forests are not uncommon in spiritual meditation. Included in this experience can be art, poetry, and music. Meditation can lead to this place for a short period.

The spiritual world can impact your life deeply in many ways. Once you experience the spiritual world in meditation, you can have a deeper awareness of a higher realm, no matter what your religion is. You may understand the real meaning of love and selflessness.

If you have an awareness of the spiritual world, death is not as scary. In meditation you can learn about the spiritual realm, thus becoming acquainted with a beautiful, wonderful place where you can be with loved ones! There is nothing to fear. When we meditate and learn about the spiritual world, death can lose its power to cause fear.

The spiritual world has been described in many ways. Some believe it is within and others believe it is distant. Each religion has its own separate beliefs about the spiritual world; however, there are many things in common with all of the religions.

Joseph Campbell (1904-1987), who I mentioned before, was a famous writer and teacher who traveled widely, studying the world's religions. He was friends with many of the great spiritual teachers of his time. He wrote brilliantly on the common threads that he found in all the world's religions. He points out the common connections between the holy days and religious rites that are important to each religion, for instance. Many holy days and religious rites have a history that predates the originator of that religion. Campbell and others have made study of the common practices of the world's religions much easier. It may be that there is only one spiritual source that is described in different ways with different ways to reach that source.

Meditation provides a tool to reach the spiritual realm ourselves without the requirement of belonging to a particular religion. This realm can be reached whether you are meditating at home or present in a religious setting. Spiritual meditation is often easier in a place where people have meditated previously, and it is certainly best done in a quiet setting.

There are different paths of spiritual meditation that are described. There is a path of devotion and a path of insight or knowing.

The first is the path of devotion to, and a desire for union with, a higher being. This is the path of Christianity, Judaism, Islam, some Hindus, and others. The one on this spiritual path worships and gives devotion to a higher being. One key part of this path is a need to request or pray for aid. Assistance is requested from this higher being to solve problems now and help you to later get to heaven. Many Christians, for instance, believe they must ask Jesus for help, to help them be "saved." They believe that a person can be saved by Jesus, just by turning his or her life over to him. Devotional meditation can use a religious object like a rosary, a religious symbol, or a visualization of a spiritual being. This focus helps the meditator to connect with a higher being.

Another path is that of insight, which helps the meditator to understand who he or she is. It is a path of study and personal exploration. On this path, the person will seek understanding of his or her thoughts and internal world. Through this knowledge, the meditator can gain understanding of the underlying reality of the world. With insight meditation there is a study of the layers of one's internal self, which will with time help one to understand the greater universe. Buddhists believe this will take several lifetimes to accomplish. After time and study the meditator will become awakened or enlightened and reach nirvana. This path can be taken alone, but it is easier with a teacher.

As the study of religions becomes more global, people are combining the spiritual practices of both the East and West. It interesting that it is possible to move from intellectual interest in the spiritual world to a deep inner belief or knowing of this spiritual world after meditation. Experiencing meditation on the spiritual level has been very meaningful and life changing for many. It revitalizes religious teachings. The spiritual becomes very real.

FLOW EXPERIENCE

In addition to the traditional ways of describing meditation, Mihaly Csikszentmihalyi, a famous psychologist from the University of Chicago, has identified what he calls the "flow experience," which can occur in everyday life without you consciously trying to meditate. It occurs when levels of consciousness are in harmony with each other.

The flow experience has the following characteristics: action and awareness merge; you become one-pointed; you have clear goals with immediate feedback, concentration, and focusing; irrelevant stimuli disappear; there is a loss of self-consciousness, an altered sense of time, good balance between ability level and challenge, and a sense of personal control, while it should also be intrinsically rewarding.[46]

Examples of the flow experience include enjoyable work, sports, music, art, fishing, yoga, martial arts, or gazing at things of beauty like a garden. During this period in the flow, awareness is altered so that time seems to slow. Athletes or artists describe being absorbed in the flow. The activity is usually one that has been "over-learned." Some have described it as being in the "zone." This feeling is the same one that is described by people while meditating, either with sitting or movement meditation. It seems humans, particularly children, can have the flow or meditative experience naturally without actively trying.

MEDITATION AND GROUNDING

The practice of meditation can increase sensitivity to and awareness of the external world. This increased sensitivity can be a challenge when functioning in a world that is noisy and chaotic. You can become calm during meditation and then have that calm disrupted in the everyday world. There are techniques called "grounding" and "sealing" that will help you preserve the calm in spite of external confusion.

---

46   *Flow: The Psychology of Optimal Experience.*

The simplest form of protection comes from the concept of grounding. Imagine a connection with the earth. If you are outside, it is possible to touch the earth or sit next to a tree. The whole idea is to connect mentally and physically with the earth to stabilize your energy.

There is a more sophisticated form of protection that is done by imagining that you are in a ball of light or sealed and surrounded by light. In Christian terms, you are "wearing the whole armor of God."[47] When you visualize being surrounded by light, you can protect yourself against the sometimes chaotic energy of the outer world. For example, the practice of crossing your heart, as taught by the Catholic church, is a form of sealing and protection. Other teachers suggest imagining a circle or a cone of light around us.

It is good to seal or ground yourself at the end of every meditation. At the end of meditation, picture being surrounded by a ball of white light. Make the ball of light as thick as you like. After all, it is free! This technique of being in a ball of white light also works during the day, particularly when entering a psychologically negative environment. Using your imagination to draw a great circle of light around you on the breath can be quite grounding in itself. Many people consciously surround themselves with white light before dealing with difficult people. It is possible to relax and be more confident when you feel surrounded by light.

---

47   Eph. 6:11, see also Rom. 13:12.

Another grounding technique is to think of yourself as a tree. The roots go down into the ground, the tree is supple but the trunk is strong, and the branches rise into the sunlight.

THINGS TO REMEMBER:

1. Meditation starts with moving the attention of the mind away from everyday concerns to a word, the breath, or an image.

2. There are three levels of exploration that can be sought in meditation: physical, mental, and spiritual.

3. Mindfulness and visualization are important techniques used with meditation.

4. Many find it helpful to end meditation with grounding or sealing.

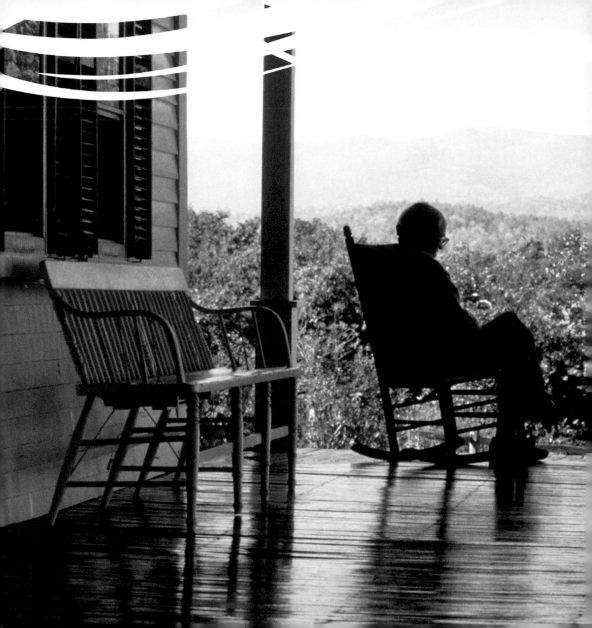

6

Frequently Asked Questions

1. How do I start?

See the chapter above. There are many ways to start meditation. You can join a class, read a book, or sit quietly for five minutes observing nature. Many people find that a quiet place, a comfortable chair, and an object to focus on are all that is needed. The support of a teacher and a class can be helpful, but is not vital.

2. Are caffeine, alcohol, or illegal drugs O.K. with meditation?

It is best to have a clear, relaxed mind when starting meditation. Unpleasant experiences can occur with illegal drugs or alcohol. Caffeine and nicotine are stimulants and can make the meditator nervous and unable to settle into meditation. Some prescription medications can also cause drowsiness and make it hard to meditate.

3. What body position is best for meditation?

For best results, sit either on a chair or on the floor. The spine should be lengthened and upright but not stiff. The sitting yoga positions including the famous (but advanced) lotus pose have been used extensively for meditation. Moving meditation, as in walking, tai chi, or yoga is also a great way to meditate. Meditation lying down is difficult, as it is easy to fall asleep; however, it will work for those who cannot be upright. The spine needs to be straight and the mind focused.

4. Is incense good for meditation?

Incense has been used in meditation and some find it helpful; however, most people choose not to use it as it can distract from the meditation. It can be unpleasant for those with allergies. For those who would like to use it, there is a guide to which incenses are helpful in the book *Incense* by Jennie Harding, uniform with this one.

5. Is it dangerous for people with mental illness to meditate?

Relaxation meditation and structured meditation (that is, with a leader) can be useful for people with mental illness. It is best for those with unstable mental illness to be treated before meditating. In any event, if there is concern, there should be permission given by a medical doctor before meditating. If relaxation is desired, there is another choice called biofeedback.

6. Is music good for meditation?

Listening to gentle music is a good way to prepare for meditation because it calms the nerves, settles the mind, and helps the meditator to focus. For most people it is best to turn off the music at the beginning of the meditation, because music itself can be distracting.

7. Can meditation become addictive?

For the great majority of us, the habit of meditation is unlikely to grow to troublesome proportions! There are reports of monks who live in seclusion either in the East or the West meditating for days, but these long meditations are not damaging for those trained to do them. There can be a temptation to allow meditation to become an excuse for not dealing with the practical issues of living. Like anything, it is best in moderation.

8. What position should the hands be in?

There are many possible positions for the hands in meditation. The most common position is with the palms up. Some people like to have their hands on their lap, with the palms up, left hand inside the right. Meditators from the yoga tradition have used different finger positions to change their meditations. They claim these positions change the flow of energy in their body.

9. Will I lose control?

You can leave the meditative state at any time you choose. The ability to enter meditation or leave meditation is like entering or leaving prayer. It is under your control.

10. Can I meditate during the day at work?

It is possible and helpful to be meditative at work by quieting the mind and concentrating attention on the work to be done. Skills learned in meditation, like being mindful, focused, and attentive can be used very effectively at work. Deep meditation is not compatible with regular work. Precaution: it is not good to meditate and drive.

11. Is meditation harmful or beneficial to my health?

Meditation is definitely good for health. By meditating, the negative effects of stressful living can be reversed. Some of the benefits of meditation include lowered blood pressure, a stronger immune system, improved breathing, and reduced atherosclerosis (a type of arterial sclerosis).

12. What can I do about the physical
distractions that occur while meditating?

It is wise to plan in advance for the meditation. Your clothing and sitting position should be as comfortable as possible without sacrificing alertness. The bladder and stomach should be empty. Caffein-ated beverages and alcohol should be avoided for several hours before meditation. Simple stretching exercises, taking a walk, or doing yoga beforehand can help settle down your body. Have a glass of water by you, especially if there is a problem with coughing; cough lozenges also may be useful.

If a muscle is tight, a good way to relax it is to tighten the muscle more and then let go. It is good to do a survey of your body, find out which muscles are tight, and relax them. Relaxing the shoulders and face is particularly important.

13. What can I do about the mental distractions that come up when I meditate?

Focusing on an object, word, or visualization will take the mind's at-tention away from the distraction. Focusing on something beauti-ful—a candle or a flower, say—is considered to take the mind away from the rational area and into the restful, creative area. When stray ideas come into the mind, it is important to let them go and then bring the attention back to the focus. Every time the attention is brought back to the focus object, it becomes easier to do. The busy mind will eventually settle down.

14. Is meditation a religion or will it interfere with my religion?

Meditation is not a religion! Many meditate who are not religious or are in non-religious settings. It has been used by many religions but it is not a religion. Meditation is a universal tool that can be used by all to develop awareness.

15. How do I explain meditation to my family?

A simple explanation of the initial meditation techniques summarized here can be useful. It may be good for you to include them in a short sample meditation. Many families enjoy meditation together. Explanation of the many benefits of meditation, including relaxation and better health, can be helpful. This book is intended to help them as much as you, so it should be a good one to lend. It is good for you to affirm that meditation is not a religion.

If your family does not meditate with you, ask them to let you have your meditation time without interruption, while being clear about the time you are going to be away from them.

16. What is a "good" meditation?

Every meditation is a good one. Concern about the quality of the meditation is itself distracting. At first, a good meditation is simply one that helps to trigger the relaxation response. A feeling of calm will develop. The heart rate and breathing will slow. Distracting thoughts will fade away and it will be easier to focus. With practice, it is possible to learn about the mind and the spiritual world if so desired.

17. How do I know I am I doing it correctly?

You or your family will begin to notice a more relaxed and calm temperament. Meditation will become easier and more fun. You will begin to see both the inner and outer world from a new perspective.

18. When should I meditate?

Any time that you will meditate is a good time. Many who have busy schedules choose to get up twenty minutes earlier and meditate at the beginning of the day. Meditation will then help the day go more smoothly. Others like to settle down to meditation after a busy day, or to use it to relax before going to bed.

19. Do clothes make a difference?

Yes, clothes should be comfortable and non-distracting with the right amount of warmth.

20. Where do I meditate?

You can meditate anywhere if it is quiet and comfortable without distractions. Phones should be off the hook so they cannot ring or be located in another room from which the sound does not travel. It is nice to meditate in the same place each time if possible. Some people have a special meditation corner or even a meditation room if the house is big enough. Just using the same chair, and maybe having a table with a candle or flower on it, is a way of building up a routine that the body recognizes, in a way that assists meditation.

21. How long should a meditation be?

Most people meditate for between five and twenty minutes daily if they are on their own. With time, and in a class, it becomes easier to meditate for longer if so desired. Meditations can last for hours or even all day. There are meditation retreats available with meditations for several days. Long meditations seem daunting but can be quite enjoyable for the experienced meditator.

22. What should my goals be with meditation?

Your goals for meditation can include learning how to relax, which is very important to reduce your stress and improve health. If you desire, you can move on to an awareness of yourself and the spiritual world. It is best not to have expectations of yourself or of your meditation as you start, however, as these are themselves distractions.

23. What are some of the big problems with starting meditation?

Finding the type or style of meditation practice you like can take a little time. When you start to meditate, learning to settle the mind and relax the body can be challenging.

24. How can I find the right length of time to meditate?

You can experiment with different lengths of time meditating and then find the one that is best for you. You will begin to feel a sense of calm and relaxation. The time spent in meditation may vary from day to day, but it is quite a good idea to choose in advance how long you will meditate for and stick to that. If you are worried about time, the worry will distract from your meditation. If you are worried about meditating too long, you can set a kitchen timer for the time you desire. A visible clock, though it means opening the eyes, may be less distracting than a fear of overrunning.

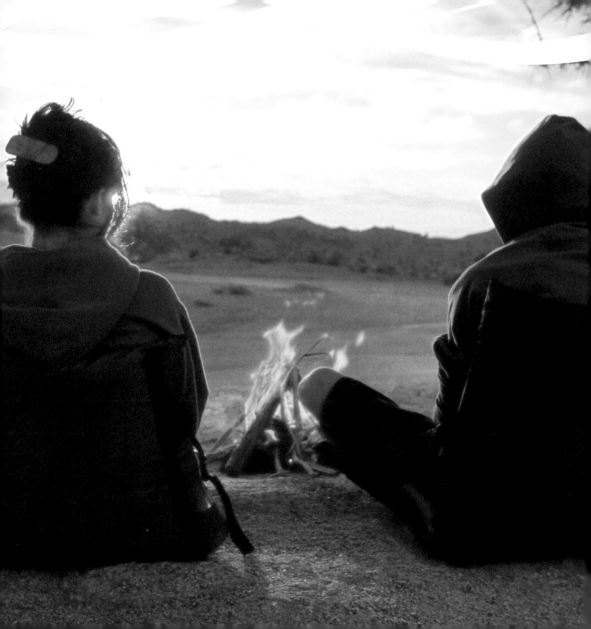

7

Sample Meditations

BEGINNING STEPS FOR ALL MEDITATIONS

- Stretch briefly.
- Have a clear mind free of alcohol or illegal drugs. (There are also legal drugs like caffeine, nicotine, and some prescription drugs that can interfere with meditation.)
- Have a calm stomach. (You do not want just to have eaten, or to be too hungry.)
- Pick a quiet, safe spot where there will be no interruptions.
- Now begin a meditation of your choice.

At the end of each meditation, take time to return to the everyday world. This is more important with deeper meditations. Some find the steps for grounding or sealing to be helpful. (See page 45.)

MINDFUL MEDITATION ON THE BREATH

Begin with slow, deep breaths. They should not be forced, but natural instead. Breathe through the nostrils if possible, and let the breath come and go easily. With the "outside eyes" closed, use the "inside eyes" to focus on the breath. Observe what the air feels like. Is it cold or warm? What does the chest feel like when you are breathing? Does the stomach move up and down? Keep watching the breath for several minutes until a sense of relaxation occurs. When distracting thoughts enter the mind, let them go. Don't think about the stray thoughts or fight them, just bring your attention back to the breath. At first, there will be many distracting thoughts, requiring a return to the breath many times. The number of distracting thoughts is not important. What is important is bringing the attention back to the breath. You can, without too much practice, meditate for ten or twenty minutes just by focusing and observing the breath.

For those who want to further pursue breathing meditation, yoga has a large body of knowledge on this subject. *Pranayama* is the study of the controlled breath and its effects on the energy of the body. Earlier I mentioned *Light on Pranayama*, a book by B. K. S. Iyengar, the famous Indian yoga teacher. It gives extensive instruction on different ways to breathe and the effects of each different type of breathing. Yogis report that this practice is very rewarding. Many yogis spend hours daily doing this type of meditation on the breath.

MINDFUL MEDITATION ON A WORD, AFFIRMATION, OR MANTRA

With this meditation, a word or affirmation is used for a focus, instead of watching the breath. Any word will do; the words "love" or "one" will work well. Repeat the word continuously, out loud or in your heart, as you wish. Let the mind focus its attention on the word. When distracting ideas arise, let them pass by and bring the attention back to the word that is being used. Some Christians like to use a phrase from the Lord's Prayer as a mantra. This meditation can be done for ten or twenty minutes or longer if desired.

Affirmations can be repeated and used as a focus instead of a single word. Affirmations should be positive and start with the words "I am" or something very similar.

Illustrations of such affirmations include:

I am calm.
I am love.
I am peace.
I am relaxed.
I am strong.

VISUALIZATION MEDITATION

This technique can be used by individuals on their own or in led-group meditations. With the latter, the leader can describe the object to be visualized, and the group then visualizes the object together with the leader, helping to deepen the meditation. Group meditations are strong because there is the power of combined thought on one thing. There are books of visualization ideas in the bibliography.

VISUALIZATION ONE

Begin to visualize a previously chosen object: a beautiful one such as a flower, jewel, or nature scene. It is helpful to describe the object in your mind. (For example, if a flower is chosen, what color is it? How does it smell? What shape are the petals? Is there dew on the flower? Can you feel the sun shining on the flower?) With continued visualization of the object, you can move more deeply into meditation. If you like, a different beautiful object can be selected for each new day you meditate.

VISUALIZATION TWO

After relaxing, visualize a beam of light shining from above, from a star or the sun. Imagine yourself moving along this beam of light until you come to a lighted door. Go through this door to a spiritual world that is shining in the light. Imagine indescribable beauty. There may be beautiful gardens, lakes, mountains, or forests. There could be beautiful buildings or temples. Animals are frequently present. These animals can come up to you for petting, even animals that in the everyday world are dangerous. Birds can land on your hand. You may find this world inhabited by spiritual beings, and these spiritual beings may be helpful in some way. You sense, perhaps, someone who has died. It can be reassuring that a loved one is as close as a meditation.

VISUALIZATION THREE

Visualize a beam of light from a star or the sun entering your body. This beam of light is centered on your heart. The light feels warm and loving. Feel the warmth and light spread throughout your body, bringing healing to all parts of your body. This light or love can then shine out from the center of your heart to people that are close to you. The beam of light can fill you (like filling a gas tank, only it is your light tank), and you can then send the light out to others all over the world. This is a simple meditation to send love to the world, something practiced by many different religions.

A variation on this meditation is to imagine a ball of light forming in front of you. The ball of light then moves into your heart. From there you send light to your body, to those around you, and then to the world.

This is a very good meditation in terms of the feelings you generate, which will be helpful in all your practice. It should be done slowly to allow you to sense the light during each step of the meditation.

MEDITATION ON THE MIND: INSIGHT MEDITATION

This meditation starts with awareness of the physical sensations from your body. This is a good way to start insight meditation, because these sensations are more concrete and easier to be aware of in meditation. Become aware of your breath going into your lungs. Is it cold or hot? Does it feel good? Then notice the hands and/or feet. Are they warm or cold? Any sensation from the body can be examined this way.

After becoming comfortable with the observation of your sensations, you can begin by observing your thoughts. Naming or labeling your thoughts will allow you to observe what you are thinking and begin to learn who you are. The next step is to explore deeper into your mind by asking questions about a given thought. Here's an example. For the thought, "I feel fat today," ask, "Why?" (Do I eat too much? Do I like being overweight? Is there a benefit to being overweight? What can I do about my weight?) You might then move on to observe your reactions to why feeling fat prompts precisely the questions it does, and so on. This technique helps you to look at the layers of deep thoughts that underlie the original thought. This is somewhat like peeling the layers of an onion. Please refer to some of the more detailed books on insight meditation mentioned in the text and bibliography.

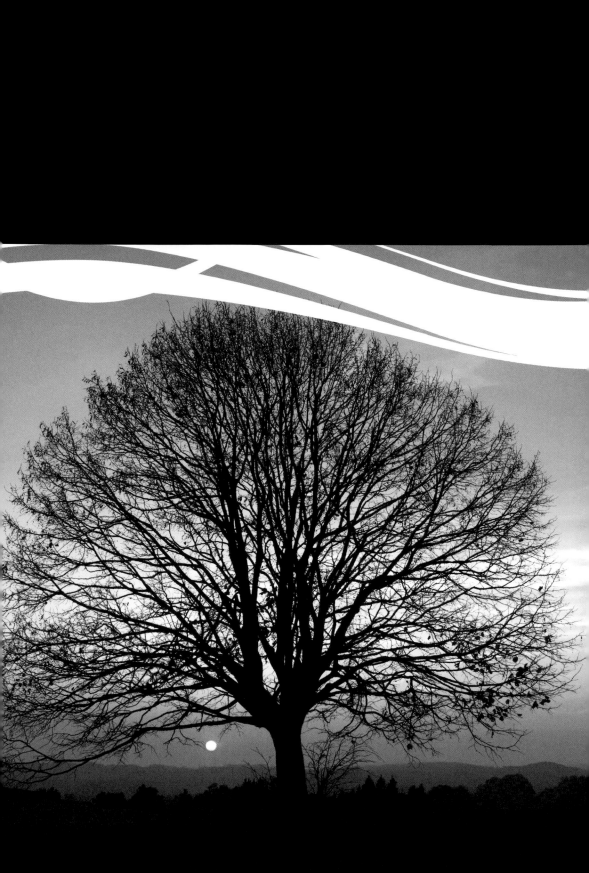

8

Effects of Meditation

ONE OF THE SIGNIFICANT BENEFITS of meditation is a greater sensitivity to beauty in the world surrounding you, the world of sounds and colors. After becoming experienced in meditation, it is possible to appreciate the world in a new way, as though in glorious Technicolor rather than black and white. Your life can become more enriched with awareness of the world's beauty.

As there is increased awareness of the inner and outer world in meditation, it is possible to understand art and music on a new level. Music concerts can be more enjoyable, and so can art exhibitions. The colors in gardens and nature settings can become more intense and beautiful. Unexpected pleasures are found in new and previously overlooked places. As consciousness expands, creative abilities may be released that were hitherto unknown.

ENERGY FIELDS OF THE BODY AND MEDITATION

The Eastern meditation traditions describe a subtle energy that is in and surrounds the body and tell us how it works in the body. It is *qi* or *prana*, the life force. There are differences between the Chinese and the Indian descriptions of the energy. Both Chinese and Indian meditation teachers, however, agree on the basic premise: that the body has a subtle energy field and it is critical to life.

Scientists have had difficulty in accepting the concept of a subtle energy field around the body, because it is hard to measure. There are many studies underway to evaluate the presence, or at least the effect, of this energy field. There are medical doctors and nurses in the field of complementary medicine who are working on "energy medicine." They believe that when a person's energy is not balanced, the body can become diseased. This is the same theory that is taught by the Eastern religions. They believe that having a body with healthy energy is the best defense against disease. Although definite proof of this theory is awaited, there has been early anecdotal evidence of the effectiveness of this approach.

Until there is more hard science, the description of the energy fields will have to come from human observers who are sensitive to seeing or feeling the human energy field. The generally accepted name for the energy field is the aura. The aura surrounds the body and extends outward several inches. The aura, according to those who can see it, is composed of different colors. Artists frequently depict an aura around the heads of saints or holy people.

People who are sensitive (those who are called psychic or clairvoyant) describe this energy or aura around the body, and they also refer to centers of energy inside the body called chakras. They are centered on the following points in the body.

1. Base of the spine
2. Pelvis
3. Solar plexus
4. Heart
5. Throat
6. Brow
7. Top (crown) of the head

There is also reported to be a flow of energy up and down the spine and spiraling around it.

Psychics claim they can see these centers of energy when they look at a person. The centers have various colors that may suggest to the observer the health of the person. Light, bright colors are said to be healthier than dark, muddy colors. As a person grows spiritually, the chakras appear to shine brighter. Artists frequently depict Jesus and other holy persons as having not just a halo, but a shining heart center as well. Krishna and Buddha are also depicted radiating light.

The concept of energy is important to meditation, although, as we have seen, it is not essential to it, except when spiritual meditation is sought. There is a large body of meditation literature devoted to energy and how to improve its circulation in our bodies. There are many types of meditation that are reputed to improve energy flow. Teachers in Eastern traditions like yoga, tai chi, and qi gong as well as many others teach about increasing the flow of energy through the body during meditation. Indian tradition has a similar concept of *prana* or life force. Either sitting or movement meditation are thought to increase and align the energy for the person doing the meditation. People describe how good their body feels after yoga, tai chi, and qi gong. They describe a sense of relaxation, but they also describe a sense of increased energy. The purpose of many of the movements is to help both the physical body and the energetic body to become balanced.

Acupuncture, which has been proven to work scientifically for chronic lower back pain,[48] works on the energy channels (meridians) in the body as described by the oriental teachers. They teach that blockages in the meridians prevent healthy energy flow, leading to pain and illness.

Meditation helps us to relax the body, clear the mind, and make spiritual connections. It has the potential to improve our well-being and balance our energy.

---

48   Lazar et al., 2005.

BENEFITS OF MEDITATION

Stress reduction and improved health are proven benefits of meditation. Many people are leading very stressful lives today and do not know how to relax. This high stress level contributes to a large number of stress-related diseases. Meditation can teach us how to move from being stressed to being calm, and it can lower the risk of disease. With practice, it is possible to maintain this calm even when under stressful conditions. The ability to reduce stress is reinforced with daily meditation.

By meditating, we can learn about who we are and what and how we think. Quiet contemplation without the noise of life will allow one to follow the ancient maxim, "Know thyself." We can learn how to improve life and find inner strengths upon which to draw. We become less affected by adverse changes in the external world. We will develop the strength to "keep on keeping on."

Experiences during spiritual meditation may teach us that we are part of a larger spiritual universe that is within and all around. The spiritual experiences can be very moving, providing a feeling of closeness to the spiritual realm.

Children benefit greatly from meditation. Recently it was reported in the *Los Angeles Times*[49] that meditation can help kids focus. "Students who've learned to meditate in school say they've learned to control their emotions before tests

---

49   Conis, 2005.

and big sporting events, even during fights with parents and siblings, by simply pausing and slowing their breathing. Fourth-grader Vanessa Macademia says the technique relaxes and refreshes her," says the report. "With research on meditation in children yielding largely positive results, some schools are using meditation techniques to treat or prevent common emotional and psychological disorders that can be barriers to learning, such as anxiety and attention deficit disorders." Meditation has helped kids improve their grades and behavior. They are using meditation as a tool to help cope with the many demands of growing.

SUMMARY OF THE BENEFITS OF MEDITATION

PHYSICAL EFFECTS

- Stress reduction
- Lowered blood pressure
- Reduction in atherosclerosis
- Improved rate of healing after surgery
- Lowered cholesterol
- Improved immune system, reducing infection risk
- Increased thickness of the brain, reversing effects of aging
- Increased neurotransmitter release in the brain, improving mood

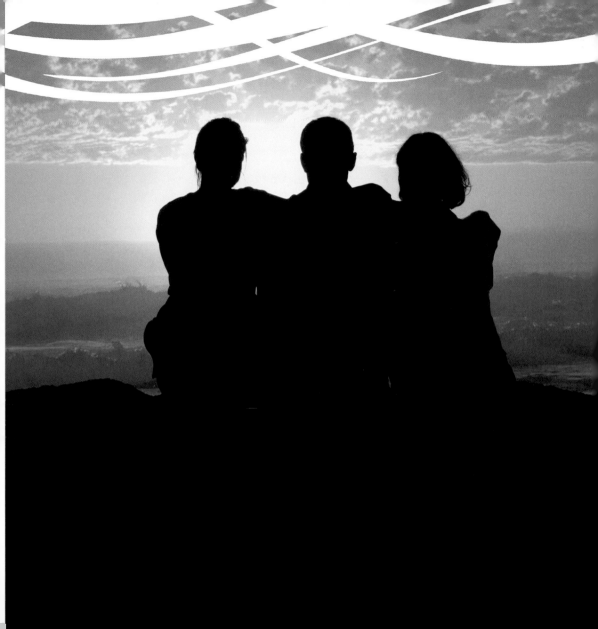

9

Why Meditation Works

MEDITATION WORKS BECAUSE it helps you to experience the seen and unseen world in a new way that is different from the mundane world. Meditation is something out of the ordinary. Meditation will raise your consciousness, helping you to gain a larger perspective of life. It offers you an enhanced appreciation of every moment of existence. The meditation experience helps you understand there is more than just the everyday world.

The meditation experience lets you look into your own mind and learn who you are. With a new awareness of self, you have the opportunity to grow and improve. Along with this new awareness of self, there also comes a greater appreciation and understanding of other humans. You can be more sensitive to the needs of others. A new perspective of the world may develop. It is easier to appreciate other religions and cultures after studying their meditation styles.

In meditation, you can learn the concept of mindfulness. Meditation teaches you how to be mindful of your surroundings. The world is suddenly full of beautiful things that were overlooked before. The world is now displayed in brilliant hues rather than black and white. Colors are more vivid, and music is melodic and rich. Interpersonal relationships may improve with your increased sensitivity to the needs of others. You become less self-centered and more aware of others. While experiencing mindfulness, there is a reduced need to be rushed. Time slows down and there is less stress produced. Every moment seems richer.

You can observe and learn about your mind in meditation. You learn that it is possible to study your thoughts. The mind has many layers. In meditation you can find out who you are and why you act the way that you do.

Meditation works to open the door to the spiritual world. This spiritual world becomes real to those who meditate regularly. In this world, you can expand your consciousness and learn to move away from the little self. Meditation on the spiritual world affirms there is ongoing life. The fear of death starts to go away. The reason for life becomes clearer.

After meditation on the spiritual realm, you can look into the future beyond death and see that there is more to life than what can be seen daily.

You too can meditate. It is not hard. The many benefits of meditation can be yours right now with a little time and effort. Now is the time to make a commitment to start meditating.

ARTICLES CITED

Benedetti, Fabrizio, Helen S. Mayberg, Tor D. Wager, Christian S. Stohler, and Jon-Kar Zubieta. "Neurobiological Mechanisms of the Placebo Effect." *The Journal of Neuroscience* 25, no.45 (November 9, 2005): 10,390–10,402.

Castillo-Richmond, A., R. H. Schneider, C. N. Alexander, R. Cook, H. Myers, S. Nidich, C. Haney, M. Rainforth, and J. Salerno. "Effects of stress reduction on carotid atherosclerosis in hypertensive African Americans." *Stroke* 31, no. 3 (March 2000): 568–73.

Conis, E. "It's cool to be calm." *Los Angeles Times*, September 5, 2005, Health section.

Cromie, W. J. "Meditation changes temperatures." *Harvard University Gazette*, April 18, 2002, pg 2.

Davidson, R. J., J. Kabat-Zinn, J. Schumacher, M. Rosenkranz, D. Muller, S. F. Santorelli, F. Urbanowski, A. Harrington, K. Bonus, and J. F. Sheridan. "Alterations in brain and immune function produced by mindfulness meditation." *Psychosomatic Medicine* 65, no. 4 (July-August 2003): 564–70.

Glaser, R. "Stress-associated immune dysregulation and its importance for human health: a personal history of psychoneuroimmunology." *Brain, Behavior, and Immunity* 19, no. 1 (January 2005): 3–11.

Gross, C. R., M. F. Kreitzerm, V. Russa, C. Treesak, P. A. Frazier, and M. I. Hertz. "Mindfulness meditation to reduce symptoms after organ transplant: a pilot study." *Advances in Mind-Body Medicine* 20, no. 2 (Summer 2004): 20–9.

Kabat-Zinn, J., L. Lipworth, and R. Burney. "The clinical use of mindfulness meditation for the self-regulation of chronic pain." *Journal of Behavioral Medicine* 8, no. 2 (1985): 163–90.

Kabat-Zinn, J., E. Wheeler, T. Light, A. Skillings, M. J. Scharf, T. G. Cropley, D. Hosmer, and J. D. Bernhard. "Influence of a mindfulness meditation-based stress reduction intervention on rates of skin clearing in patients with moderate to severe psoriasis undergoing phototherapy (UVB) and photochemotherapy (PUVA)." *Psychosomatic Medicine* 60, no. 5 (1998): 625–32.

Kiecolt-Glaser, J. K., T. J. Loving, J. R. Stowell, W. Malarkey, S. Lemesho, S. L. Dickinson, and R. Glaser. "Hostile marital interactions, proinflammatory cytokine production, and wound healing." *Archive of General Psychiatry* (December 2005): 62.

Kiecolt-Glaser, J. K., D. Ricker, J. George, G. Messick, C. E. Speicher, W. Garner, and R. Glaser. "Urinary cortisol levels, cellular immunocompetency, and loneliness in psychiatric inpatients." *Psychosomatic Medicine* 46 (1984): 15–24.

Kjaer, T. W., C. Bertelsen, P. Piccini, D. Brooks, J. Alving, and H. C. Lou. "Increased dopamine tone during meditation-induced change of consciousness." *Cognitive Brain Research* 13, no. 2 (April 2002): 255–9.

Lazar, S.W., C. E. Kerr, R. H. Wasserman, J. R. Gray, D. N. Greve, M. T. Treadway, M. McGarvey, B. T. Quinn, J. A. Dusek, H. Benson, S. L. Rauch, C. I. Moore, and B. Fischl. "Meditation experience is associated with increased cortical thickness." *Neuroreport* 16, no.17 (November 2005): 1893–1897.

Miller, J. J., K. Fletcher, and J. Kabat-Zinn. "Three-year follow-up and clinical implications of a mindfulness meditation-based stress reduction intervention in the treatment of anxiety disorders." *General Hospital Psychiatry* 17, no. 3 (May 1995): 192–200.

Neimark, J. "Impertinent ideas: alternative medicine pioneer Candace Pert." *Psychology Today* (November–December 1997).

Newberg, A., A. Alavi, M. Baime, M. Pourdehnad, J. Santanna, and E. d'Aquili. "The measurement of regional cerebral blood flow during the complex cognitive task of meditation: a preliminary SPECT study." *Psychiatry Research* 106, no. 2 (April 2001): 113–22.

New York Times. "Hypnosis." November 11, 2005, Science section.

Ornish, D., L. W. Scherwitz, J. H. Billings, S. E. Brown, K. L. Gould, T. A. Merritt, S. Sparler, W.T. Armstrong, T. A. Ports, R. L. Kirkeeide, C. Hogeboom, and R. J. Brand. "Intensive lifestyle changes for reversal of coronary heart disease." *Journal of American Medical Association* 280, no. 23 (December 1998): 2001–7.

Padgett, D. A., and R. Glaser. *Trends in Immunology* 24, no. 8 (August 2003): 444–8.

Peng, C. K., I. C. Henry, J. E. Mietus, J. M. Hausdorff, G. Khalsa, H. Benson, and A. L. Godberger. "Heart-rate dynamics during three forms of meditation." *International Journal of Cardiology* 95, no. 1 (May 2004): 19–27.

Riskes, R., M. Ritskes-Hoitinga, H. Stodklde-Jorgensen, K. Baerentsen, and T. Hartman. "MRI scanning during Zen meditation: the picture of enlightenment?" *Proceedings of the International Conference of the Transnational Network for the Study of Physical, Psychological, and Spiritual Well-Being* (July 2002).

Sapolsky, R. "Sick of Poverty." *Scientific American* (December 2005): 92–99.

Specca, M., L. E. Carlson, E. Goodey, and M. Angen. "A randomized, wait-list controlled clinical trial: the effect of a mindfulness meditation-based stress reduction program on mood and symptoms of stress in cancer outpatients." *Psychosomatic Medicine* 62, no. 5 (2000): 613–22.

BOOKS MENTIONED IN TEXT OR RECOMMENDED FOR FURTHER READING

Barnes, Martina Glasscock. *The Meditation Doctor*. Hauppauge, NY: Barron's Educational Series, Inc., 2004.

Beeken, Jenny. *Don't Hold Your Breath*. London: Polair Publishing, 2004.

Benson, Herbert. *The Relaxation Response*. New York: Avon Books, 1975.

Bodian, Stephan. *Meditation for Dummies*. Indianapolis: Wiley Publishing, 1999.

Cooke, Grace. *Meditation*. 4th ed. Liss, Hampshire, England: White Eagle Publishing Trust, 1999.

Csikszentmihalyi, Mihaly. *Flow: The Psychology of Optimal Experience*. New York: Harper & Row, 1990.

Fontana, David. *The Meditator's Handbook: A Complete Guide to Eastern and Western Techniques*. London: HarperCollins,1992.

Gawain, Shakti. *Creative Visualization: Use the Power of Your Imagination to Create What You Want in Life*. Novato, CA: New World Library, 2002.

Goldstein, Joseph, and Jack Kornfield. *Seeking the Heart of Wisdom: The Path of Insight Meditation*. Boston: Shambhala Publications, 1987.

Goleman, D. *The Meditative Mind: The Varieties of Meditative Experience*. New York: Tarcher/Putnam, 1988.

Hanh, Thich Nhat. *Peace is Every Step: The Path of Mindfulness in Everyday Life*. New York: Bantam, 1991.

Harding, Jennie. *Incense*. London: Polair Publishing, 2005.

Iyengar, B. K. S. *Light on Pranayama*. London: HarperCollins, 1992.

Kabat-Zinn, Jon. *Full Catastrophe Living: Using the Wisdom of Your Body and Mind to Face Stress, Pain, and Illness*. New York: Dell, 1990.

Kabat-Zinn, Jon. *Wherever You Go, There You Are*. New York: Hyperion, 1995.

Mack, Gaye. *Making Complementary Therapies Work for You*. London: Polair Publishing, 2005.

Mishra, Pankaj. *An End to Suffering*. Basingstoke, England: Picador, 2004.

Monaghan, Patricia. *Meditation: The Complete Guide*. Novato, CA: New World Library, 1999.

Murphy, Michael, and Steven Donovan. *The Physical and Psychological Effects of Meditation*. 2nd ed. Sausalito, CA: Institute of Noetic Sciences, 1998.

Myss, Caroline, Ph. D. *Anatomy of the Spirit*. New York: Three Rivers Press, 1996.

Ornish, Dean. *Dr. Dean Ornish's Program for Reversing Heart Disease*. New York: Random House, 1990.

Pert, Candace. *Molecules of Emotion*. New York: Scribner, 1997.

Rinpoche, Sogyal. *Meditation: A Little Book of Wisdom*. London: Rider, 1994.

White Eagle. *The Still Voice*. Liss, Hampshire, England: White Eagle Publishing Trust, 1981.

Wilhelm, R. (trans.). *The Secret of the Golden Flower*. London: Arkana, 1988.

THE NURSING MOTHER'S HERBAL

SHEILA HUMPHREY, BSC, RN, IBCLC

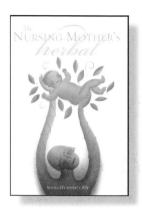

Which herbs can a new mother take to increase or inhibit milk production? Are there natural remedies for mastitis or chronic yeast infections? This integrative guide answers these and other questions about the effects of herbs, dietary supplements, and other natural products on nursing women and their babies.

Sheila Humphrey is an RN and Lactation Consultant in a hospital-based practice, and is a La Leche League Leader.

ISBN: 978-1-57749-118-7 • $16.95 pbk • 6 x 9 • 355 pages

Published in cooperation with the Center for Spirituality and Healing, University of Minnesota.

Fairview Press

2450 Riverside Avenue South, Minneapolis, MN 55454

(800) 544-8207 • www.fairviewpress.org

KARMA AND HAPPINESS

A TIBETAN ODYSSEY IN ETHICS, SPIRITUALITY, AND HEALING

MIRIAM E. CAMERON, PHD, RN
WITH A FOREWORD BY HIS HOLINESS THE DALAI LAMA

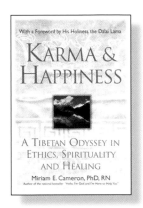

Karma and Happiness explores the connection between ethical behavior, spiritual practice, and physical wellness. Part travelogue and part inner journey, the book chronicles the author's journey to Tibet and her personal search for a more complete spiritual and ethical framework.

ISBN: 978-1-57749-105-7 • $16.95 pbk • 6 x 9 • 272 pages

Published in cooperation with the Center for Spirituality and Healing, University of Minnesota.

Fairview Press
2450 Riverside Avenue South, Minneapolis, MN 55454
(800) 544-8207 • www.fairviewpress.org

PATHWAYS TO SPIRITUALITY AND HEALING

EMBRACING LIFE AND EACH OTHER IN THE FACE OF A SERIOUS ILLNESS

Alexa W. Umbreit, ms, rn, chtp
and Mark Umbreit, phd

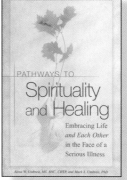

A mind-body-spirit guide to coping with serious illness—written for patients and those who love them. Provides an overview of modern methods of self-healing, advice on confronting death and loss, healing meditations from seven different faith traditions, a list of resources, and a glossary of terms.

ISBN: 978-1-57749-110-1 • $14.95 pbk • 6 x 9 • 160 pages

Published in cooperation with the Center for Spirituality and Healing, University of Minnesota.

Fairview Press

2450 Riverside Avenue South, Minneapolis, MN 55454

(800) 544-8207 • www.fairviewpress.org